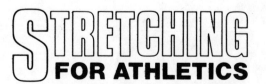

GOLD
DIGGERS OF
1929

Contents

Preface to the Investment Classics Edition

In the past few years, several new American books have testified to people's abiding fascination with the terrible financial calamity that, while it did not cause the Great Depression, at least contributed to it and certainly announced its beginning. *Rainbow's End: The Crash of 1929* by Maury Klein (Oxford University Press, 2001) is doubtless the most readable of these. During the same period, a work of Canadian scholarship has devoted considerable attention to Canada's own version of the Crash, which was simultaneous with the U.S. one but differed in essential ways. This is *Blue Skies and Boiler Rooms: Buying and Selling Securities in Canada, 1870-1940* by Christopher Armstrong, published by the University of Toronto Press in 1997. All this while, *Gold Diggers of 1929* (the title is a play on the names of such Depression-era Hollywood movies as *Gold Diggers of 1933*) has remained in print almost continuously, much to the astonishment of its author.

I wrote this essay on the 1920s (for that is essentially what it is) to suggest how much modern Canada was shaped by the decade in question. That was, after all, the period when the country moved from being a rural society to an urban one and the economy started to extend significantly beyond agricultural and resource production. It was also the time when, having stood upright on its own in the Great War, Canada began to question its place in the British Empire, if not yet to wax so anxious as it has done subsequently about the American empire that supplanted it. It was then that Canada asserted its own culture. As much as the 1920s were about jazz or Prohibition, they were also about, for example, the Group of Seven. These statements have become clichés because they are so true.

The book was published in 1979 to coincide with the 50th anniversary of the Crash. Its admittance now to the Investment Classics series comes during the 75th anniversary. When I was writing it, there were still many people alive who had suffered in the Crash as adults. There were even some who had been important in the Canadian investment field of the time; I was privileged to be able to interview a number of them. Today there can be no such personal nostalgia. On the contrary, perhaps what new readers will find of interest in the story is how impossibly remote it seems from their own experience of Canadian business life.

Such shifts in memory and perception were of course already quite far advanced when I was writing the following pages, though in the 1970s it was still possible, just barely, to recognize in this particular past the origins of the present. Since the last time I wrote a preface to this text 15 years ago, however, change has accelerated so quickly as to make the tale sound like the ancient history it is— and therefore (he says hopefully) to hold out a different sort of attraction to another generation of readers.

The Toronto Stock Exchange (TSE), which is at the centre of this study, has never shied from putting new technologies to work. The TSE wasn't the first exchange to install stock tickers. Significantly, though, it was the first to include actual sales prices, rather than merely bid-and-asked quotations, on its ticker tapes. Similarly, it didn't assist at the birth of the digital age, but it did install, in 1977, the first computer-assisted trading system (CATS), though it took another 20 years for the TSE to end floor-trading entirely. Since then of course various descendants of Toronto's original CATS have become ubiquitous round the world. The universal nature of such software helps point to other even more significant developments. Who would have expected then that Leningrad (as it then still was) and Shanghai would soon have vigorous stock markets to raise capital for their countries' restructured economies? Or that, as part of the same process of realignment, Canada's regional exchanges would have to reposition themselves or perish? The feeling was that for capital markets to become global (as seemed to be the trend, for better or for worse—or both) they must first become truly national.

In 1929, Bay Street in Toronto still had not overtaken St. James Street in Montreal as the country's financial centre. Montreal's suffering, however, began not long afterwards. By 2001, when the Montreal Stock Exchange got out of the stock-trading business after 127 years to reinvent itself as a derivatives market called the Bourse de Montréal, no one was surprised, for the institution had long been in steep decline. The energy was moving westward not only to Toronto but beyond. In 1999, the Vancouver and the Alberta exchanges joined together under the name Canadian Venture Exchange and soon consolidated operations with the TSE's Canadian Dealing Network or CDNX. The Winnipeg exchange at first refused an invitation to join but later relented after admitting that continuing on its own was impractical. By that time, the CDNX already had acquired the junior listings of the Winnipeg and Montreal exchanges. Later, the TSE was renamed the TSX and the Venture Exchange became the TSX Venture Exchange, on which about two-thirds of the TSX's 4,000 or so companies were listed.

Applause for the way such moves created a national structure for small-capitalization companies to raise money seemed to drown out concerns about the loss of local and regional autonomy, small-c cultural as well as economic. For example, a proud tradition of almost uninterrupted chicanery finally came to an end when the Vancouver Stock Exchange, which *Forbes* once described as "polluting much of the civilized world," finally sacrificed its existence to national interests. Readers of true crime are directed to *Fleecing the Lamb: The Inside Story of the Vancouver Stock Exchange* by David Cruise and Alison Griffiths (Douglas & McIntyre, 1987).

In 2002, the TSE demutualised and went public as TSX Group Inc., the type of fundamental change that the New York Stock Exchange and the Nasdaq had only contemplated now and then. As one commentator pointed out, by becoming a virtual marketplace the exchange had in a sense returned to its roots, when there was no big board and a small group of wealthy investors met to trade shares among themselves. Except that the old boys were gone now. In a sense, the process had been democratized.

All this makes the environment sketched in *Gold Diggers of 1929* seem all the more remote and unbelievable but also, I hope, even more remarkable for its strangeness.

GF, Vancouver, 2004

Preface to the
Original Paperback Edition

In September 1920 someone tried to destroy Wall Street by setting off a gigantic bomb in the middle of it, killing thirty people and wounding several hundred. The *New York Times*, like the rest of the press, suspected that anarchists or Bolsheviks were behind the explosion, which it called "a piece of organized devilry executed with a terrible effectiveness. . . ." But no one was ever arrested for the crime, even though individuals as far away as Hong Kong tried to confess, hoping that they would be extradited to the United States and thereby avoid the usual immigration formalities. At one point in the investigation, however, the evidence seemed to point to Canada.

It came to light that a Toronto resident named Edward P. Fischer, who previously had been employed in the New York financial district, had sent postcards to his former colleagues, warning them of some terrible disaster. "Keep away from Wall St. the Wednesday after next," read one of the communiqués. "There never was a road that did not have a turn." At length, the authorities were forced to dismiss Fischer as an eccentric and the timing of his messages as so much coincidence. Edward Fischer was soon forgotten, and that seems a pity, for he is a useful symbol of the historic

connection between the U.S. and the Canadian stock exchanges—
as well as of the crucial differences that unite them in a web of
volatility, linked to the ups and downs of the two economies as well
as to the greed and fear of the investing public.

This little book was written in 1979 on the 50th anniversary of
the great stock market crash of 1929. My aim was not simply to look
at that event from a Canadian perspective but actually to reclaim
something unmistakably Canadian that had been misplaced in the
rush of popular history. There was, and is, a tendency to suppose
that the crash is one of those events that is so American in character
as to be a wholly American phenomenon. It was widely believed that
what took place on the Canadian side of the border was merely a reaction to it or a faint imitation. But just as the settlement of the
Canadian west followed a totally different course from that of
the American west, or just as, so Pierre Berton reminds us, the
Klondike gold rush was in essential ways a different type of occurrence from the California one, so too was the Canadian crash of
1929 not separate but distinct from the American.

Proportionately, Canadian speculation in U.S. securities was if
anything more extensive then than it is today, but even that long ago
the dynamic of history was clear. Canada was in a transitional period, when British capital and political influence were giving way to
American. In that breathing-space between dynasties, however,
Canada was able to maintain some economic dignity. Yet for a variety of reasons, which I tried to address in the following pages, the
crash in Canada was in fact worse than the one in the United States,
worse because Canada was so much more vulnerable to such events,
and worse certainly in the severity of what it presaged. It was a terrible catastrophe for the Canadian economy, but at least it was
Canada's own catastrophe. It was negative proof of economic— "in-
dependence" is not the right word, but perhaps "distinctness" will
do. Some type of natural self-image not only survived it but, by
doing so, became more clear. A lesson of the same sort is perhaps
the best souvenir of the crash of October 1987 as well.

Given the way that the world's population is always growing, life and society are themselves, so to speak, inflationary. Hence it is misleading and dangerous to assume that there is a correct relationship between yesterday's figures and today's. Some words I used in this book only 10 years ago, such as when I referred to the historic plateau of one thousand for the Dow Jones Industrial Average or guessed at the number of millionaires in Canada, seem terribly dated today; the fact that now, in 1988, there are seven Canadian billionaires near the top of the *Forbes* list of the world's wealthiest people probably will seem just as antiquated a decade from now. In view of such change, it is impossible to know what to make of the 1987 crash, which wiped out nearly one trillion dollars in paper wealth around the world, except to say that although it was bigger than the 1929 crash, and even more international in scope, it was less serious, because it did not lead directly to the world-wide depression so many people were expecting.

What happened was that on Monday, October 19, there was an enormous wave of panic selling in New York, where the Dow Jones fell 508.32 points, or more than 22 per cent. A record 604 million shares were traded: enough to sorely test, but not, as in 1929, to actually break, the exchange's capacity for recording them. In Toronto, the TSE 300 Composite dropped 11.3 per cent; in Montreal, the Portfolio Index, 9.53 per cent. When the exchanges closed in the United States, people waited for the panic to strike the other markets around the world. The *tsunami* hit Tokyo first, cutting the Nikkei Stock Average, then Hong Kong, where trading was suspended part way through the day, then Sydney, where the All Ordinaries took a drubbing.

Many observers were quick to blame the crash on programmed trading, in which computers were used to execute volume trades automatically at certain price levels; others pointed to the increasing number of funds indexed to stock prices themselves, or to any of a number of other causes. Whether or not they admitted it, everyone seemed to know what the underlying factors were: extraordinarily high debt levels, particularly in the United States, which had a national debt of 2.3 trillion dollars at the time, and other such imbalances which also bespeak the global nature of the economy. For all the interdependence through technology, however, and despite the realization among the investor class that they are playing in one vast polyglot market linked by satellite, there was no world-wide financial meltdown. For a time at least, people seemed to eschew the idea that stock market movements are portentous in themselves. They returned to an older notion that such calculations are merely a barometer, albeit a wild barometer, of corporate performance and of social and economic health, an instrument for measuring present reality and short-term expectations. Appearances to the contrary, they seemed to be saying, it was not yet, or not any longer, an engine of universal Americanism. To that small extent, there was still, amid the gloom, a little hope for Canada.

GF, 1989

1

The Crash and the Depression

Winston Churchill was wearing a funny hat. The future prime minister of Great Britain was touring Canada, and between public and private engagements he found time to indulge his favourite hobby, painting. He sat on the terrace of the Banff Springs Hotel creating a landscape of the Bow Valley. He was dressed in the floppy, brimless piece of headgear and long linen duster he always wore at such times. A few days later he would push on to Vancouver to open the annual fair of the Royal Agricultural and Industrial Society of British Columbia with some encouraging words about the nation's economy. "We see Canada," he would say, "growing in every way—education, civilization, numbers, and wealth." That was on September 3, 1929, the day the Canadian and American stock markets reached their absolute pinnacle. The next day they developed a serious crack as a result of the speculative boom which is so much a part of what we conjure up when thinking of the 1920s.

This breach should have been a warning to the Western economy that the bull market of the past few years had grown too large, that the sky-high prices must, by the laws of economic gravity, come plummeting down. It should have been, but it was not. Few people interpreted the slip in stock prices as much more than a momentary bit of turbulence, and then in the following months the entire system collapsed.

The worst day was October 29, 1929, known ever afterward as Black Tuesday, though Thursday of the previous week (Black Thursday, October 24) had first signalled the end. Just as before nothing could shake investors' optimism, now nothing could contain their panic. On the Montreal Stock Exchange that day, 500,000 shares were unloaded, or five times the usual traffic. On the Toronto Stock Exchange, where 25,000 or so was the normal volume, the transactions totalled 330,000 shares. The exchange floors were in pandemonium. Traders could not begin to keep up with the selling orders that poured in, and the Morse ticker machines which carried the latest prices fell hours behind. On the New York Stock Exchange, a staggering 16 million shares were sold in what was quickly recognized as the worst single day in American financial history. An anxious, uncomprehending crowd gathered outside the building, like the peasants who, in movies yet to come, see a light in Castle Frankenstein and mill around it with pitchforks and torches. Inside, the gallery had to be closed and the visitors removed. Among the spectators ushered from the building was Winston Churchill, still on his North American jaunt.

Some economists have suggested that Churchill was really to blame for the Crash of 1929, at least to the extent that he was responsible for the boom. Their reasoning is that Churchill, after becoming Baldwin's chancellor of the exchequer in 1924, returned Britain to the gold standard, or rather, to the pre-Great War relationship between gold, the pound, and the dollar. The pound was thus overvalued, and this led to the first of Britain's periodic exchange crises and contributed greatly to the 1926 general strike. But it also pointed, more immediately, in 1925 and again in 1927, to demands by Britain, but also by Germany and France, for easier credit from the United States. So the Federal Reserve jiggled the rediscount rate, at which its member banks might borrow. The foreign governments purchased U.S. securities, which put a lot of cash into the country, and this money went directly to the purchase of stocks or to people borrowing for that purpose. The result: the greatest bull market ever known and, perforce, the greatest crash. Until evidence found in his papers showed he had the decision forced on him by the City and the Bank of England, the notion cherished by many economists was that Churchill had returned the pound to its pre-inflationary position on little more than a romantic impulse. It was thought that he never understood the consequences, which included 10-per-cent unemployment for Britain through most of the 1920s, just as John Maynard Keynes had forecast.

This assessment was fairly sophisticated all the same and was made with hindsight by persons familiar with economic theory. It is thus in contrast to most other pat answers that came on the heels of the events themselves, as the markets dipped still lower in November and reached absolute bottom in 1932, amid the worst days of the Depression. These were the times when, to take one dramatic Canadian example, the stock of Abitibi Paper, which had traded at $35 at one point in 1929, sold for only 13 cents. Immediately following the Crash and for a long time afterward, everyone was blaming everyone else for the debacle. Some ascribed guilt to Sir Joseph Flavelle, who still suffered from a bad press stemming from wartime allegations, never proved, that his company, a precursor of Canada Packers, had engaged in profiteering. In November 1928, another company he controlled, Canadian Marconi, shot up from $4 to $28.50 on the old New York Curb Exchange despite the fact its earnings were sometimes only a penny per share. Flavelle said in an interview in the *Financial Post* of Toronto that he thought the price much inflated; within 48 hours the shares fell to $8 in New York, igniting a brief panic estimated in one account to have cost billions in share values.

But Flavelle wasn't the villain. Nor was Arthur W. Cutten, another Canadian, thought by some to have played bear on the bull market on such a scale as to rupture the machinery of speculation and net himself millions. These people and others like them may have been factors, though they were less important than a credit system that allowed speculators to purchase stocks on as little as 10-per-cent margin, a system that remains the stock culprit in simplistic schoolbooks on the period. But the real scoundrel was greed, avarice, the get-rich-quick psychosis which overtook a remarkably wide spectrum of the North American population in the years following the hitherto unparalleled destruction of the First World War. It was an unpleasant characteristic within ourselves, one not lessened by time, that led to the Crash and the still worse developments later.

The Crash did not create the Depression that followed it. Although there is still scholarly debate on the exact cause and effect, the best learned opinion is that the Depression would have happened anyway; indeed, that it would have happened even without the connivance in the early 1930s of Mother Nature, which lent horrific overtones to the very word Saskatchewan. The economy was overproducing phenomenally in the 1920s, and in such circumstances there is never a gradual realignment or a graceful winding-down. The Crash was the inevitable coupling of the boom and the gloom; if it hadn't come on Black Tuesday, it would have fallen on some other day of the week, some month or other, if not in that year then the year afterward, and made it just as dark in the consciousness of an entire generation. Yet for all that it was the single most disastrous occurrence in the era between the wars. And more than most other cataclysmic events, it is surrounded with mythology.

When the stock market collapsed, brokers and investors committed suicide by jumping out of windows. This is one myth about the Crash, and it began taking hold at once. Stories about falling bodies circulated in New York even as the events unfolded, and within days jokes about it began appearing in the press. In one of them, a man asks a hotel desk clerk for a room and the clerk replies haughtily, "Will that be for sleeping or for jumping, sir?" Another warned visitors to New York to beware of falling bodies when walking in the

vicinity of Wall Street. The facts, however, do not support the existence of a period when it rained bulls instead of cats and dogs.
Some old-timers still swear it happened, but the stories are often
contradictory. In the newspapers, which then often reported suicides as suicides, the evidence is even weaker.

In his book about the American crash, written on the 25th anniversary in 1954, John Kenneth Galbraith pieced together statistics
showing that, both nationally and in New York, the suicide rate had
been climbing throughout the 1920s but that the last months of
1929 were no worse in this respect than any other time. The sharp
increases were in the early 1930s, when the Depression was in its
stride. But there's no evidence to suggest that a noticeable proportion of even these deaths was related to current events, though the
chances are better that many in fact were the result of financial
woes. But then, too, the economic situation seemed to provide an
easy answer to what is always an unanswerable question: why?

Rumours about men on high ledges were probably given credence by several well-reported suicides in the financial community
carried out by other means. In an irony equal to Edgar Rice
Burroughs' dying while reading the funny papers, the president of
the Rochester Gas and Electric Company took his life by inhaling gas.
In early November, J. J. Riordan, a prominent figure in Democratic
Party circles in New York and the president of the County Trust
Company, shot himself with a revolver he had taken from one of the
tellers' wickets; the story was big news despite the efforts of political friends, including New York's governor, Al Smith, to cover up.
Smith was also accused, in 1932, of intervening in a similar manner
after Ivar Kreuger, the Swedish match king, shot himself in Paris. But
these were the primary incidents.

Writing on the 40th anniversary of the Crash, Alexander Ross
in the *Financial Post* found Canadian figures similar to Galbraith's.
He cited 1926, if not as the peak year for stock market prices, then
the year in which investor confidence was highest (the Canadian
Marconi incident being still in the future). The suicide rate that year

was only 7 per 100,000 people. The figure rose in 1927, fell in 1928, then climbed to a peak of nearly 10 per 100,000 population in 1930 and continued at almost that level through 1932. Here, apparently, there were no well-publicized instances of financiers doing themselves in—only an incident in which a disgruntled Montreal stockbroker took a potshot at Canada's most powerful businessman, Sir Herbert Holt. Says Floyd Chalmers, who was then editor of the *Post* and later the president and chairman of the Maclean-Hunter media empire, "I never had any friends who jumped out of 10th-storey windows."

Americans who had been wiped out, then, were not engaging in wholesale defenestration. There were, however, the other dramatic deaths so conspicuously absent here, which may help account for a more important and ultimately more dangerous myth about the events of 1929. *In Canada, the Crash wasn't so severe as in the United States* runs a widely held belief. The idea is that the economy didn't crash here so much as it slid, in a kind of toboggan ride to desperation. On any chart of market activity in the two nations, the giddy ascendant lines and the terrible ones of decrescendo must inevitably correspond. But this fact doesn't supplant the presumption that, like our own western settlement alongside that of the United States, matters were quieter and more orderly this side of the border, and so the Crash was an obviously less important turning-point. This is another view at variance with the facts.

As a sign of what was to come, the Crash was the classic instance of a cold in the United States manifesting itself as pneumonia in Canada, and for this reason alone it deserves to be remembered. Few if any industrial countries, even the States, were harder hit by the Depression than Canada was. At one point in May 1933, unemployment passed the 32-per-cent mark. That was the worst single year, when the Gross National Expenditure was only 58 per cent of what it had been in 1929. But the real difference among nations was not in the severity but in the longevity of the crisis. In Britain, for instance, the Depression was long and bleak enough, though cynics would say a keen eye was necessary to distinguish the 1930s in this regard from the troubled 1920s. The Depression exaggerated the economic polarity inherent in the social structure, but by 1935 or so the worst was long over. In the United States, conditions got better quickly when President Franklin Delano Roosevelt, coming to office in March 1933, took matters in his own hands and instituted a brace of daring government relief and work programs. In Canada, R. B. Bennett's Conservatives had defeated the Liberal government of Mackenzie King in the 1930 general election and set about working on the problem. First they tried boosting imperial trade. Then they tried "blasting" Canada into world markets. Finally, the Tories turned to their own version of the New Deal. But the scheme was later found by the Privy Council to be unconstitutional; the economic system on which the country operated may have made it unworkable anyway. Canada's economy was then dominated by others just as it is today.

The arguments are by now familiar to all, but in 1930 they had not assumed quite the full stature of ideology. The sheer size of the country, the small and thinly spread population, and the nature of its industries all meant that great infusions of capital were necessary to maintain the standard of living which Canadians, who were quickly leaving the countryside for the cities and towns, had come to expect. This capital came from outside. In 1930, non-residents owned 40 per cent of the manufacturing and 56 per cent of the then still all-important steam railways. Canada was an exporting nation owned to a great extent by its customers, who naturally managed to sell us more than they acquired. In 1928, we sold 38 per cent of our exports to the United States but purchased 67 per cent of our goods from the south. With Britain, the figures were stacked in the other direction (they bought 22 per cent of our exports and we imported 16 per cent of what we needed from them). But in basic ways this was no more reassuring. Nearly half of our exports were in base metals, wood and forest products, wheat, and some other areas of agriculture. These were the fields in which (along with the fisheries industry, especially in the Maritimes) we naturally took the worst beating. In some cases we had been over-producing these anyway. In 1928 record grain yields were reported and wheat sales were very depressed. It was also then that we achieved world dominance in newsprint (formerly known as paper). But in this area, too, a glut was obvious. When world trade took a nosedive, we were carried down along with it, and being so tied to the health of other nations could not recover as quickly as the rest.

At least this was the major factor. But our hands were tied in other ways as well. Canada had experienced a quite severe recession after the First World War. It was the first in which Ottawa gave money for unemployment relief to the provinces, which in turn channelled it through the municipalities. One way out of a recession was spending on railways. So much money went into construction that in 1923 the federal government amalgamated many small, half-completed lines only to find that the new combined venture, the Canadian National, had a debt of more than $800 million even before it started. By the time of the Crash, the settlement of the West was complete, wheat was already king, and railway construction was practically saturated, but the government was still carrying the enormous costs.

Now Ottawa had to come to grips with the two traditional courses of action in any depression. The first was spending on public works. By the early 1930s, however, the provinces and cities were already doing this; in fact, they had been borrowing for this purpose so that they, too, had over-extended their credit. The second response was to squeeze credit in order to force out speculators and, in a fit of Calvinist glee, make them suffer. To some extent, Ottawa did in fact do this, imposing a sauna-like atmosphere after a long period of national debauch. But the built-in rigidity of the economy was simply too great.

Our internal economic and political machinery, however, did leave us at least one certain advantage over the Americans in terms of recovery. It was inevitable, for instance, that the Crash, caused partly by easy credit the speculators could not resist, should practically destroy the credit system in the United States in the early years of the Depression. By 1928, the States, with its entrepreneurial tradition, had more than 31,000 banks, some of them capitalized on as little as $100,000 or perhaps even $75,000. Regulation was minimal by today's standards, and the range of their activities wide. The banks were permitted to lend on industrial mortgages, for instance, unlike the monolithic chartered banks of Canada (in those days there were ten of them). The panic brought wholesale runs on the banks, and as many as a third of them folded before Roosevelt imposed a moratorium in 1933.

In Canada the credit system was far stronger. Except for issuing bank notes, the banks then were essentially as they are today. There was no instability on the American scale. The Home Bank of Canada, which had collapsed in 1923, was the last major casualty. But then Canadian banks were essentially commercial institutions, with no involvement in consumer loans and residential mortgages. Indeed, when the banks did move into consumer loans it was only by means of chattel mortgages, and until relatively recent times they were limited to charging 6 per cent on loans. To the bank manager of only 25 years ago, today's practices would have seemed imprudent at best, if not downright bohemian.

None of this, however, could mitigate substantially the agonizing slowness of Canada's recovery. As late as 1937, government and consumer spending had recovered to 1929 levels but investments and the all-important exports remained way down, and the Gross National Expenditure was still an obstinate 13 per cent below pre-Crash figures. It's axiomatic to say that normalization would have come in time even without the Second World War to stimulate industry and agriculture, just as the Depression would have taken place even without the Crash. But it's also true that for Canada, of all countries, the European conflict couldn't have come too soon so far as the economy was concerned.

2

Gold Diggers and Mudhens

In 1933, Americans were singing a tune about the disappearance of breadlines and threatening landlords. It was originally called "The Gold Diggers' Song" when written for the film *Gold Diggers of 1933* but became popular under a title taken from the refrain, "We're in the Money". At that stage, the optimism of the lyrics still contained a great deal of wishful thinking but such was America's public face at the time ("Happy Days Are Here Again" had been Roosevelt's campaign song only a few months earlier). Although Canadians sang along, in that rockbottom year, they had much less reason to take the words literally. Anyone looking into the events preceding the Crash, however, would do well to consider the implications of the song as a piece of popular culture reflecting the mood of the times.

Except in movie titles, the concept of the gold digger, or amatory entrepreneuse, has not survived very well the nostalgic revisionism by which later generations sift through the 1920s, keeping some images, letting go others. The gangster, the Babbitt, and the flapper have remained integral parts of what most people think of when the decade is mentioned. But the gold-digging showgirl or starlet, like the lounge lizard, the sheik, the flagpole-sitter, and the marathon swimmer, has not lingered in quite the same way. This is a shame in a way, for she remains a useful symbol of a social attitude then at its most prominent; she is at the very heart of the *other* 1920s, the one the expatriate writers and artists of the period were running away from in disgust. She is the symbol of materialism run amok in an age when wealth, at least paper wealth, was more easily available and more fervently sought after by the populace at large than at any other time before or since.

The boom in the years after the First World War, and the fear of politics and mortality the war had suddenly aroused, went together to create what might be called a gold-digger society. If the phrase thus applied comes only in long retrospect, the usefulness of the gold digger was even then apparent to some commentators in the confused period immediately following the Crash. On Black Tuesday, the *Toronto Daily Star* carried a report from New York on the mood of gloom in the "leading gouge emporiums" and other expensive night-spots. "During the entire stretch of this bull market," the story stated, "New York has been the gold digging capital of the world.... One may safely estimate that the beautiful Lorelei Lees from Paris, Vienna, Buenos Aires, Madrid, Muscatine, Iowa, and Flatbush sluiced more millions out of these diggings than the forty-niners got out of Sutter Creek. Up until a year ago, they ran two and sometimes three shifts, and the takings were stupendous." In 1930, one of the feature syndicates supplied newspapers with a similar story; it took the form of doggerel purporting to express the thoughts of a typical gold digger. The verse began:

What's all this talk of Hoover holdin' meetin's every day?
What's this I hear of business needin' aid?
What's all the line of chatter about trouble on the way
And hints about no money bein' made?
I dunno what it's all about—my readin's very slight—
At headlines I have only taken peeks;
I had a sort of feelin', though, that somethin' wasn't right
For no one's sent me orchids, oh, for weeks!

It concluded:

> I s'pose I ought to keep in touch and know just what is what,
> And why it is and when it is and how;
> I hate to think I'm not a very well read person, but I've simply
> been too busy up to now;
> I know that somethin's happened, though, that must be pretty
> tough
> And I'll just quiz my "daddy" till he squeaks;
> He can't fool me no longer with his "Nothing wrong, dear" guff—
> He hasn't sent me orchids now for weeks!

The popular picture would have it that such true gold diggers were inadvertently smarter than most of their fellow citizens in that they probably kept their money in jewels and furs presented as gifts, and cannot, as a professional group, be presumed to have speculated on the market. But this leads to another of the deceiving myths that have sprung up about the late 1920s: that everybody and his aunt was playing the market. In reality, the speculation, though staggering, was less widespread than the mania for it.

There can be no doubt that all the financial centres were witnessing what insiders called a mudhen market, in which thousands of totally unqualified speculators, all hoping to cash in, succeeded only in driving up prices and overloading the circuitry. That much at least was obvious by the volume of trading, though figures on the exact number of such naïfs were never tabulated. Rather, the press, in scrambling for colour reporting to lend the news a human emphasis, made the stock market a popular topic everywhere.

One Toronto paper, for instance, discovered that elevator operators in a downtown skyscraper were ruined after forming an informal consortium to play the market. In another story, a prominent city bootlegger was rumoured to have lost $200,000 in cash. Certainly the range of people gambling in securities extended further down the socio-economic scale than is now customary; one could judge this by the crowds of secretaries and other office work-ers choking the brokerage offices during the lunch hour. But the harshest fact about the Crash is that it decimated, not the once-in-a-lifetime crap-shooters and the widows and orphans, but the solid middle class.

The Crash may have shaken the entire society with a terrible new sort of tremor—the realization that if big corporations could suddenly tumble, then nothing and no one was safe. But its main immediate effect was in clobbering the middle-income business-men, managers, and professionals who were the backbone of the society, economically at least, and who never let you forget it. Here, too, the exact numbers were never available. Some measure of this sector's strength, however, can be gleaned from the fact that, according to the *Daily Star*, the events of October and November were estimated to have cost $12 million to a total of 35,000 Torontonians in various walks of life, about 6,000 of them women. That was a sizeable chunk of the population in a city of just over 600,000. It did not represent the entrenched old moneyed fami-lies—they muddled through, as they always had done—but was made up instead of what today would be called the upwardly mo-bile. A good illustration of the difference is to compare the effects of the Crash upon the personal fortunes of Mackenzie King and two later prime ministers.

King didn't play the market. He had no need to do so. After los-ing his House seat in 1911 he made a nice living as an industrial relations consultant to such figures as John D. Rockefeller (who once gave him a gift of $100,000) and Andrew Carnegie. Then, in the early 1920s, a Liberal businessman named P. C. Larkin, later president of Salada Tea and (at the same time) Canada's high com-missioner to London, began a non-partisan fund for King, as benefactors once had done for Macdonald. He raised $225,000. On Black Tuesday, King gave the first of his staid little pep talks on the country's economic state. It is perhaps significant, however, that as events were unfolding he made no mention of the Crash whatsoever in his famous diary. His kind, if they weren't too terribly cautious, saw the battered bull market as a sign that they could pick up certain stocks cheaply in the times ahead.

R. B. Bennett was a different sort, a truly wealthy man who had made his fortune in business, or rather, in his case, had had it handed to him. In 1921, he inherited controlling interest in E. B. Eddy Limited from Eddy's widow and one-time nurse. He saw no reason to dispose of it when he became Conservative leader in 1927. "I am not at the moment making any disposition of my shares in the Eddy company," he wrote at the time to Colonel John B. Maclean, the Toronto magazine publisher, "but I have received two offers and the sale price would run into several millions of dollars."

The spectacle of the prime minister owning the giant Eddy company, whose log-jams in the Ottawa River were visible from his Centre Block office, might seem an inexcusable conflict of interest today. Fifty years ago, however, wealth was not considered an impediment in politics; the public, in fact, appeared to put a greater trust in leaders who were rich, perhaps because such men seemed bred for leadership and service, or possibly just because they were thought less likely to steal.

At any rate, it was an era when conflict of interest was not so meticulously defined or closely monitored as it later became, in terms of both money and power. It was a time, for instance, when the premier of Quebec, Louis Alexandre Taschereau, served on the boards of a dozen corporations, when Sir James Lougheed (Peter Lougheed's grandfather) was both the Senate Conservative leader and a lawyer for the CPR, and when the mayor of Toronto, Bert Wemp, also happened to be city editor of the *Evening Telegram*. In this atmosphere, R. B. Bennett created no scandal with his holdings, which plunged in worth when the Crash came but made him an increasingly wealthy man once more as the economy slowly recovered. He was another of the fortunate on whom the Crash had no long-term effect. In this as much as in party affiliation he differed from Louis St. Laurent.

St. Laurent was not basically wealthy. In fact, until tapped by King as minister of justice, he was essentially just another Quebec City lawyer. He did build up a handsome portfolio but was so badly hurt in the Crash that he had to take many cases beneath his abilities and was still paying off his debts during the Second World War. He was precisely the sort of person who got sucked in, he and the whole range of salesmen, middle-level businessmen, professionals, and para-professionals such as pharmacists. Being closer to the financial world, the lawyers were probably the first to return to the market after the wounds healed. But the others were scarred for years to come; untold thousands likely never went back but put what came their way afterwards into insurance and savings bonds. This was all much later, however, when the stock market had long since ceased being the glamorous, kinetic place it was in the middle and late 1920s.

In the heady days of 1929, ordinary folks discussed playing the market the same way people in 1969 spoke of scoring dope; in elevators, on trains, and at parties they bored everyone silly with talk of their portfolios the way today people do with chatter about their RRSPs. It was a mark of glib sophistication to refer to stocks by their nicknames: Monkey Ward for Montgomery Ward (the American mail order giant), Big Steel for United States Steel, Little Steel for Bethlehem Steel Corporation. On both sides of the border, having a broker was like having a bootlegger in the States—the minimum demanded of one in terms of status, like an American Express card now.

The upsurge of interest was not confined to the principal centres; a smallish city such as Kingston, Ontario, population 25,000, had four or five brokerage houses where before it had only one family-owned firm catering exclusively to the area's traditional elite. This mood was naturally reflected in the popular culture of the time. During the week of the Crash, the Strand cinema in Calgary was playing a picture called *The Wolf of Wall Street*, starring Nancy Carroll and George Bancroft. Later in the panic, Shea's Hippodrome in Toronto featured Bill Robinson and Jason Robards, Sr., in *The Gamblers*. "Wall Street," ran the advertisements, "where the greatest drama of the age is played—with its cemetery at one end, the river at the other and the suckers in between. A golden heaven for the few, blackest hell for the many."

Magazines, especially, were full of stories about individuals making fortunes in six months. The result was a blurring of responsibility, as the paper success of a few speculators aroused media fascination, which in turn increased the number of stock market gold diggers, who only brought more attention to bear on the trend, in a vicious circle. Once again, however, a distinction must be drawn between the ordinary middle-class investor, overzealous though he may have been, and the under-informed luster after the fast buck, with an eye cocked toward a new house, a fur coat, a Pierce-Arrow, a Packard, or even the ultimate, a Duesenberg. Both have to be viewed in their proper financial and physical environments, however unclear the difference between them became in the frantic motion of the times.

That people bought so many stocks must be seen, in another twisted bit of karma, in relation to the fact that there were so many stocks for them to buy: the supply increased to meet the demand as demand outstripped availability. During the First World War, many people who had never invested before got into the habit through the medium of victory bonds. Then, in the inflationary period after the Armistice, many came to view stocks as a good hedge. Concurrently, the business world changed its own attitudes toward stock issues. Earlier in the century common stocks had been given away as sweeteners with bonds, which were the main vehicle of corporate money-raising. By the early 1920s, however, common stocks were firmly established as an extremely popular form of investment in their own right. The bond market was not abandoned but neither was it where the action was. "A distinct and rather significant change has taken place in the course of investment," the Montreal *Gazette* commented editorially not long before the day of reckoning. "On both sides of the line there has been a more or less general disposition to swing away from bonds and similar securities to give a preference to stocks. The reason for this is obvious. Stocks have a speculative outlook; and speculation is today rampant throughout the world to a degree wholly unprecedented."

The action, more specifically, was not only in blue chips but in junior industrials (which often traded at up to 30 times earnings) and in a new phenomenon (new on this continent at least), the investment trusts. These were in effect pools to which one subscribed by buying shares and which in turn invested in the broader market on the members' behalf. They thus resembled today's mutual funds except that they were closed-end; that is, they issued a limited number of shares. To the man in the street who wanted his slice of the good life they seemed an almost ideal instrument. Instead of tying up his little lump of capital in a few shares of one or two companies, he could put the money into a trust whose supposedly astute analysts would select, on behalf of all such purchasers, the best issues at any particular moment. This new idea, the capitalist co-operative, had been prominent enough in Britain for years; when the notion spread to North America in the middle 1920s, it was taken up with incredible enthusiasm.

In the United States, choosing a trust was almost as complicated as playing the market *without* the middleman. In 1929 alone, some 265 so-called trusts were established, though many of these were in fact holding companies, trading corporations, and speculative companies of one sort or another. The Americans even set up several trusts for the sole purpose of investing in the shares of Canadian banks—six of which, to meet the growing demand for loans and to maintain suitable reserves, had issued almost $39 million worth of stock. In this as in many other cases, the trusts' wholesale buying habits boosted the prices of the stocks they took an interest in.

Canada had about 40 trusts. They dealt almost entirely in domestic stocks and thus helped counter the habit of Canadians at that time of investing in foreign securities. (There are no clear figures showing how much Canadian money went to Wall Street. It was recorded, however, that in 1929 about 60 per cent of stocks bought in Winnipeg were American as against only 5 per cent by 1951; and this is probably typical of the nation as a whole.) That was the good side of the trusts that everyone applauded. In most other ways the trusts were controversial.

Before the Crash, their defenders were saying that these trusts could prove an invaluable economic safety valve; if the market ever started to slip, the trust managers, in search of bargains but also in a kind of altruism for which no precedent existed, would pump things up by putting their weight behind issues that were falling. It was also suggested that in other times they could be used to act against inflation. But in practice, as wiser heads made clear, the trusts were a force for volatility, not stability. In many cases, with their huge assets, the trusts literally controlled the fate of sizeable corporations. At the least they tended to usurp much of the floating supply of share capital so important to the marketplace. Worse still, there was a great deal of pyramiding, with trusts investing in other trusts which had perhaps invested in still others.

That the trusts were another big contributor to the Crash is beyond doubt. That the public gobbled them up insatiably is even more clear. They may not have been the greatest thing since sliced bread (as sliced bread was still a new commodity in 1929), but some metaphor of this sort is needed to express their popularity. Trusts were unregulated almost totally and without much standardization: some were restricted to permanent investment while in others stocks could be sold off any time at the discretion of the managers; still others worked on a unit system whereby a depositor could take delivery of his stocks from a trustee only after he had purchased a certain number of units.

When new trusts were formed in New York, they were frequently sold out within 24 hours, with other prospective purchasers turned away. In the United States, they sometimes traded for two or three times their book value. Canadians on the whole were some-what more discriminating, and prices were usually at or even below book value as the Crash approached. But even so, people in Montreal, Toronto, and elsewhere were cashing in their bonds and eschewing nice safe real estate to play the game, and some of this money undoubtedly found its way to trust managers. And these, mind you, were on balance the more sober gold diggers. The wilder ones added a new dimension to the term by putting their money in mining. Many mining corporations, like most trusts, were on the square; the venture capital actually went toward exploration and ex-traction. But in countless cases investing in Canadian mining stock was a far more figurative way of throwing one's money down some hole in the ground.

3

Con Men and Suckers

Then and for some years afterward, Montreal was a far more important financial centre than Toronto, with a larger stock exchange. Montreal, in fact, was supporting two major exchanges after 1926. That was the year the Montreal Curb Exchange opened, trading shares not listed by the bigger and more staid Montreal Stock Exchange. Thus the city was following the pattern of New York, where for decades shares not listed on the primary market had been bought and sold on the sidewalks of the financial district. This custom of "curb" trading ended when the brokers of the New York Curb Exchange (now the American Stock Exchange) moved into their own building in 1921.

Toronto, too, had a curb exchange, though it was insignificant compared with the city's two main marketplaces, the Toronto Stock Exchange and the Standard Stock and Mining Exchange. All the junior exchanges in those days were associated with the occasional bit of sharp practice. But Toronto was somewhat different: its mining exchange, the largest in the world, was routinely, almost preposterously, crooked. This fact helped accelerate the trend by which Toronto finally outstripped Montreal as the leading financial city. The process, however, was basically a slow, steady one, like that by which Calgary could one day push Montreal out of the number two spot.

Montreal in 1929 was a bustling but polarized city of one million people. Impressive amounts of construction were visible everywhere, and politics were changing as quickly as the cityscape. A few months earlier Camillien Houde had been a virtual unknown. More than a decade later he would be jailed for seeming to oppose conscription. In time, he would prompt the *Toronto Daily Star* to compose Canada's most infamous headline: "KEEP CANADA BRITISH / DESTROY DREW'S HOUDE / GOD SAVE THE KING." But as the Crash neared he was just beginning the first of his many terms as mayor, and would leave briefly to lead the Conservatives in the provincial house. Economically, it was a time when the banks were expanding their power, when the boom in manufacturing was at full throttle, and when the fur-trader days seemed farther in the past than they actually were. "It was at once Liverpool and Lombard Street, Pittsburgh and Wall Street," Stephen Leacock, who still taught political economy at McGill, would write one day. It was the country's economic nerve centre because it was the country's largest city, and vice versa.

The Montreal Stock Exchange was formally established in 1874, though its roots go back much earlier. It began with only 63 issues, 21 of which were bank stocks. Next in order of volume came bonds and debentures, railway stocks, and then industrials. Only 3 of the 63 were mining companies. The city had come a long way since then in terms of industrialization, and other events helped rearrange such percentages as these. But the original list is still useful for illustrating where the Old Money came from and where it was kept. It creates a pretty staid picture of the Montreal financial world.

Not that Montreal wasn't a hub of sometimes ill-informed speculation; it was, in most ways, the epicentre of the general market boom. The number of stock transactions per year rose from

4 million in 1925 to 19 million in 1928, the price of an MSE seat from $27,000 in 1921 to $225,000 in 1929. But several factors made Montreal less conducive to obvious chicanery.

For one thing, the line between rich and not so rich ran parallel and very close to the line between linguistic solitudes. Enormous chunks of the city's power were wielded by the wealthy anglophones scattered about the mountain. The old Montreal under-writing houses such as Nesbitt Thomson, Greenshields, and Royal Securities were perhaps even more conservative than the generally newer Toronto ones (A. E. Ames, Dominion Securities, and Wood Gundy), which would in time surpass them. In Montreal, it was not unusual for a senior partner or frequently even the president of such a brokerage to spend all day watching the board and phoning an end-less succession of Westmount patriarchs, recommending they buy this and sell that. The financial community was run essentially by people who were members of (in descending order of exclusivity) the Mount Royal Club, the Mount Stephen Club, and the St. James Club. In all three dining-rooms, Gallic names were unusual except on the printed menu cards.

There were, of course, rich French-Canadian families and indi-viduals with some hand in the business of securities (they belonged to the St. Denis Club), but many fewer than today. At the mudhen level, there simply was not the sort of mass speculation among francophones that there was, in Montreal and elsewhere, among English speakers. Certainly there wasn't the interest in semi-rural and small-town Quebec that there was in similar parts of other provinces. Money went instead to locally owned Quebec savings banks and to caisses populaires. Also, in a great many communities it was customary to trust one's money to the district notary to in-vest on one's behalf. Ancestral memories, it seemed, remained strong. Twice French Canadians had been stuck holding bad paper money—in the last year of the Conquest, and during the American invasion of 1775-76, when American money was forced on them. They didn't care to be burned yet again.

This reluctance may have been one reason why Montreal was a less tumultous place than Toronto at the time. The other reason was Toronto's almost complete domination of mining activity in the eastern half of the country. It was customary in the 1920s for Toronto brokers to spend two or three days a week in Montreal, buying batches of securities to peddle back home. But in mining, Toronto was the focal point for the whole of North America. It was also the centre of stock fraud, for the two seemed to go together. The hub of such behaviour was the Standard Stock and Mining Exchange, whose members were estimated to have bilked $100 million from 400,000 customers during the gold-digging years.

The Standard was a long four-storey building on Richmond Street, a discreet distance from the more sedate senior exchange on Bay. It had been formed in the 1890s and fed on the Klondike rush, but it came into its own in 1903 when the world's richest silver deposit was found at what is now Cobalt, Ontario, a town that sprang up willy-nilly around the discovery site. The Yukon experience was only a few years old and the mass hysteria it produced not quite ready to die. Excitement ran even higher when, within a short time, a chain of other discoveries (gold for the most part) were made at such places as Red Lake, Porcupine, and Kirkland Lake. A full-scale boom was on. It tapered off soon enough to the status of a steady, important Ontario industry growing phenomenally each year from 1922 to 1929. But it remained a boom and not a business in the imaginations of suckers everywhere. There were indeed many legitimate fortunes created overnight. For example, Edmund Horne, who discovered Noranda, made millionaires of 13 of his buddies in New Liskeard. But a great deal of money was also to be had preying on foolish investors.

Once the rush had peaked there rose up around Canadian mining a whole subculture dedicated mainly to chicanery. Many of the victims were Americans who tended to picture Canada as a frontier where fortunes could be made by lone individualists with hardihood enough to battle the elements. But many of the perpetrators were also Americans: penny-stock hucksters who poured into Toronto escaping the so-called blue-sky laws passed in the United States with just their sort in mind. The Yankee whisky traders of the West may be better known to history but they hardly match these modern-day bandits for perniciousness and colour.

Phoney mining promotions were not the only scam. One favourite con (it had several variants) entailed keeping a watch on the newspapers for the obituaries of company directors. Spotting such a notice, the bunco artist would option the stock. Then he would call on the bereaved widow, introduce himself as a casual associate of her husband, and offer to ease what must be her pressing expenses by purchasing the dead man's shares. While she pondered the offer, a night letter would arrive from a still closer associate. It would warn her that she might be contacted to sell but should resist the urge as new internal developments affecting the share value were about to be made public. By the time the first man returned to hear her decision, greed would have done its work: the woman would end up buying the stranger's own holdings at a much inflated price. He and his confederate at the telegraph office would then slip back across the border until matters cooled.

By no means a majority of the scoundrels were from the United States, however. But quite a few Americans joined the Canadians who got themselves accredited as members of the Standard (sometimes despite their criminal records) and went into business as bucket-shop operators.

I remember one fellow [recalls Floyd Chalmers] who used to sell circulation for the *Financial Post*. He wasn't very good at it. Anyway, he left us and began to peddle mining maps on the Street. Then he ran into another person who had no background in brokerage, and the two of them set up a firm and within eighteen months they were living very high on the hog. I remember going to see them in about January of 1930 and they had this great big office just filled with period furniture.

He had four telephones, one in each corner of the room, so wherever he happened to be he could just reach out and use one of them. I remember I went to a big party he gave one time at his house down near the lake south of Oshawa. It didn't take them long to start spending money as though they were millionaires, which they were. On paper.

The map-seller eventually served two and a half years in penitentiary, less time off for good conduct.

Canadian mining in this period was not dominated by big money, international connections, and geophysical science. It still depended on grubstakers and sourdoughs. The quintessential racket involved some young go-go broker purchasing, for perhaps $15,000 or so, the unproved but legally filed claim of a down-at-the-heels prospector who may or may not have been on the level himself. A company would then be chartered and several million shares issued. A $25,000 balance in the treasury and a promise to sell 10 per cent of the stock publicly were enough to meet the Standard's listing requirements. The broker and his fellows in the Standard would then begin boosting the price by dubious means. Often this meant nothing more than planting stories in the Toronto newspapers, all of which then had mining editors. Sometimes even more serious financial publications would be induced to stretch the truth or at least put it in the most optimistic language possible. Thousands of prominent men let their names be used on prospectuses, and an engineer could usually be found to attest to the limitless potential of the site, the engineers in that time having no strong professional watchdog association. If necessary, a mine could even be salted with ore samples from another operation.

Such outfits were known as boiler-rooms when they involved the use of high-pressure sales techniques, especially salesmen with braces of telephones in unmarked rooms somewhere. The classic stock market con, however, was the simplest: the old-fashioned bucket shop in which brokers pocketed funds received from their customers instead of executing orders. But by the late 1920s this procedure had become less common in the face of police crackdowns—and because exchange members could do better through a more sophisticated type of bucketing.

The Toronto Stock Exchange in those years had at least one bucket-shop operator as a member. It also had a few members who also had seats on Richmond Street. But once again the majority of scoundrels belonged only to the Standard. They would solicit business from speculators, who would open margin accounts and begin issuing buying orders. The broker would purchase at least some of the stock in question, usually about 30 per cent, but withhold the majority of the funds put up on margin. He would then go short on his own customers, betting against them that the shares would plummet. The client would receive confirmation of his transaction. But as a margin trader, he had no right to demand delivery of the stock certificates until and unless he paid his full balance. Jack Hammell, the Toronto-based mining magnate and the most important individual in the legitimate mining industry, ran advertisements in the newspapers advising purchasers of stock in his own company to demand delivery. But few were in a position to do so.

When an individual did decide to ante up and quit the game, or when he was sold out by a broker for failing to put up more margin, he would find his holdings had been sold at the day's lowest figures. Almost invariably, of course, they had been acquired originally at the day's high. Thus the broker made an extra little gravy even from those token customers he was not cheating wholesale. "For the speculative public," Floyd Chalmers would write in his memoirs, "it was like a horserace in which the public sold its pari-mutuel tickets at a profit before the race was won. The race was fixed and the 'winning' horse was to break a leg or drop dead just before the finish line was reached."

The anti-fraud section of the Criminal Code was the only avenue of redress for investors foolish enough to deal with other than an old-established brokerage house. A few provinces did pass securities fraud laws before the Crash, but the laws weren't tough enough to clean up the business. There were, in any event, practically no investigators with sufficient training to carry out the work, and no securities commissions to do it for them. Municipal police would sometimes take an interest in the problem, but only occasionally and fleetingly. In September 1929, for instance, the Vancouver police began looking into bucketing on the notorious Vancouver Stock Exchange, which was also heavily occupied with mining. But they dropped the matter without taking any action.

Securities, then, and mining stocks particularly, were traded in an almost laissez-faire atmosphere in so far as the law and self-regulation were concerned. Historically the job of exposing the most outrageous wrongdoers had fallen to the press, though the press itself was not always above reproach. The single great exception until this time was *Saturday Night* under the reign of Charles Frederick Paul.

It was Paul, the editor from 1909 until his death in 1926, who established the famous "Gold and Dross" feature, a review column for stock issues, which later editors continued. He was an American who had come to Canada as a newspaperman not long after the turn of the century, and he attacked the financial charlatans with the vigour of a crusading frontier editor. "On page six of this issue," he wrote in a typical moment, "will be found a full account of the launching of Canadian Estables, Limited, which stands to-day as unquestionably the most bare-faced swindle ever perpetrated upon the Canadian public. Without a dollar, without a visible asset, these men, who deserve the attention of the police officers, were able here in our own Godly Toronto to load upon the public a concern which never should have been granted a charter, much less have passed the inspection of the Provincial Secretary's Department." Although *Saturday Night* had some effect earlier in the century, in the 1920s it was the *Financial Post* that cleaned up the Street and embarrassed the powers that be into enforcing the law. The ironic twist is that it did so after the Crash, which wiped out so many of the harebrained speculators upon whom the Standard and other junior exchanges had a special dependence.

The *Post* had been founded amid the recession of 1907 as a financial weekly devoted to Canadian content exclusively; not until 1968 did it begin running quotation tables from the New York Stock Exchange. This policy also put the *Post* at a distance from its nearest rivals, the *Financial Times* and the *Monetary Times*, the second of which was to a great extent concerned with insurance. The *Post* of those days was largely an investment paper rather than a more general business one. Allowing everything for the typographic gulf that separates us from the 1920s, modern readers would still not find it easy to digest. But the paper's legend and its reputation both got a big boost under Chalmers, who joined it as a reporter in 1919 and became editor in 1925, when he was 27. It was he who wrote, though with no byline, the 10-part series of muckraking articles about the Standard which appeared between November 1929 and the following January and which contributed to the eventual arrest of 27 stockbrokers, many of them millionaires.

The stories were not the same in tone as investigative journalism of a later day. They did not, for instance, name names; they offered no hard evidentiary information that could lead to charges against anyone in particular. Also, they made no secret of the paper's bias or expectations. "Without hesitation," went the first instalment, "the *Financial Post* declares that it is time for the Standard Stock and Mining Exchange to invite the fullest enquiry into its affairs and to reveal the attitude of all members as to the practice of short selling by members which has resulted in such damaging losses to the public." Soon the demands escalated ("Nothing short of a royal commission with powers to investigate beyond the limits of one province or one country will fit the demand of the present time"). But so did the scope of the practices it uncovered.

By the second week, November 14, the *Post* went to obvious pains to let a representative broker defend short selling. "The public loses a lot of money by speculation in mining shares," the member was quoted as saying. "A lot of that money comes back to the brokers. In their hands it forms a sort of gigantic pool from which Canadian mining development is financed." But by the following week, the paper began its twofold policy of (1) printing laudatory letters from small investors, patting the *Post* on the back, and (2) using these and other means toward the ultimate goal of embarrassing authorities who were hesitant to act against exchange members.

Only the previous year, the provincial parliament had passed the Securities Frauds Prevention Act of Ontario, which did seem to enjoin "stockateers" (as they were called in an internal *Post* memo) to good behaviour. But the law lacked the teeth of a similar new statute in New York State. The Ontario legislation included the demand that stock exchanges secretly audit their members, and the TSE complied almost at once. But the Standard seemed to be dragging its feet, with some tacit understanding that the province would allow it plenty of time for internal housecleaning despite the hot breath of Chalmers on their neck. The Ontario attorney general appeared to be occupied elsewhere, investigating fraudulent muskrat farms.

By the fourth instalment, the cumulative response of investors, bankers, and editors had become as much a part of the proceedings as the articles themselves. The past president of the tiny Victoria Stock Exchange, H. E. Hunnings, was quoted as saying the "sensational disclosures ... can have nothing but a good effect on the Canadian market." The daily press was enthusiastic also, and dissenting voices in any quarter were few. The *Northern Miner*, most of whose advertising consisted of announcements for new mining ventures and stock issues, took a clubby tone. It opined as how this whole unfortunate situation "could be settled in an afternoon by the brokers themselves."

Just as there seem to have been a few bad apples at the Toronto Stock Exchange, so it appears there were good ones at the Standard. A sort of reform caucus within the organization was reportedly trying to repair the damage to their reputation. One of its tools was the blackballing of proposed new members. But the *Post* was not much impressed by their efforts, at least in practice, and continued with more and different instances of what one person called "financial atheism".

They went into some detail, for instance, about blatant insider trading. Using leaks from an unnamed Excise official in Ottawa, they also came down on washing operations. In those days, wash trading referred, as it does now, to the practice of selling shares back and forth without a change in beneficial ownership, so as to attract public attention. But it also meant the process by which a broker would distance himself from the most obvious sort of skull-duggery by investing through other houses which he himself secretly owned. This was apparently a lucrative endeavour for the decoy as well as for the true owner. Many small bankrupt broker-ages were kept afloat for this purpose and at enormous cost to the larger firms that really pulled the strings. It was even more com-mon for big brokers to secretly control other ones simply to get more orders to bucket and hence more margin money to use to their own ends.

The *Post* quoted one individual who had been in the process of purchasing a seat on the Standard when he was approached by a nefarious character. "You're crazy to tie up $100,000 in a seat," the fellow told him. "We'll do your business for you, carry all your stock with ours so that you won't have to arrange loaning facilities, and give you 75 per cent of the commissions." The newcomer re-fused. But many men, equally honest, were forced, once the bottom fell out of the market, to sell themselves in this way, prov-ing a sort of Gresham's Law in which bad houses drove out or corrupted the good.

"The *Financial Post* is not so sanguine and unsophisticated as to hope that a new deal for mining will immediately result from revelations it has made and the nation-wide interest it has aroused in the prob-lems of mining finances," Chalmers wrote in the last episode of the series, in the bleak January of 1930. "But it feels that the ground-work has been laid for a firmer, stronger structure and it undertakes constructively to add new stones to this structure as opportunity is afforded." The paper had made an unprecedented splash and had helped counter the constant stream of brokerage hype with some much needed anti-hype of its own. But still no government action had been taken against the objects of the paper's indignation. Ontario's attorney general, Colonel Billy Price, KC, was beginning to look like a slacker, especially after Alberta, Manitoba, and British Columbia started investigating their own mining brokers and the Montreal Stock Exchange began boycotting the Standard. But Queen's Park was busier than it seemed, busier at least than the *Post* knew or was willing to acknowledge, and in not too long a time the story of the Standard reached a climax.

The first sign of serious trouble came on January 11 when the Ontario Provincial Police arrested Harvey Mills in Toronto. At practically the same moment, I. W. C. Solloway was being tailed in Vancouver, preparatory to his own arrest, on orders from the attorney general of Manitoba. Solloway, who had once been a labourer in his native England, and Mills, the owner of a Buffalo cigar store, were the heads of Solloway, Mills and Company, the largest mining brokerage in the country. In time, both were tried in Calgary (where they had one of their 40 offices) on four counts of conspiracy as set out in the federal Criminal Code; the charges stemmed from their bucketing activities. Solloway was fined $225,000 and sentenced to four months' imprisonment, Mills $25,000 and one month. Both of them, however, served an additional 23 months in default of the fines. The laying of these charges was still quite a sensation when, on January 30, Toronto and Ontario police pounced on brokers with the surprise and simultaneity authorities usually reserve for rounding up radicals.

Shortly before 7:00 a.m., a team of 16 city and provincial detectives arrived at police headquarters on College Street for final instructions. By 7:45 they had arrested nine members of the Standard at their homes and were leading some of them downtown in pairs. The men, most of whom had been asleep when the detectives appeared, represented the five largest firms in mining. All were charged under Section 444 of the Criminal Code, just as Solloway and Mills had been. In fact, warrants were issued for Solloway and Mills as well, though it was understood the Alberta action would take precedence. A warrant was also issued for a twelfth man, who was in Montreal.

The nine arrested that day were not small-fry. For the record, their names were: D. S. Paterson, Malcolm Stobie, Charles J. Forlong, Austin Campbell, W. T. Shutt, James Heppleston, Maurice D. Young, Gordon Draper, and William J. Smart. The man being sought in Montreal was John W. Wray. All were released on $100,000 bail, though Smart had already posted that amount a week earlier when he'd become the first person arrested under the *Securities Frauds Prevention Act*. His firm was Homer L. Gibson and Company, which Gibson had sold to him only the previous September for $4 million before moving to California, where he led an unmolested life. More than a dozen juniors in the various firms were also taken in and held as material witnesses.

To defend them at their trial in the fall of 1930 the accused re-tained the best legal talent of the day at fees ranging up to $1,000 per day. There was a rumour that one Crown witness had been offered $50,000 to leave town and remain inaccessible, but this was never substantiated. All were convicted and served sentences of from two to three years in Kingston. Solloway and Mills were tried separately once released from jail in Alberta but pleaded *autrefois acquit* and this time were let go. In 1932, Solloway published a book, *Speculators and Politicians*, in which he defended himself on the grounds that every-one was doing what he had done. He detailed how, starting with nothing in 1926, Mills and he had built up in four years a $70 million line of business with fifteen hundred employees.

The newspapers played up the dramatic arrests in the fashion of the time with photos of the accused being led away and of their ex-pensive homes. In the *Daily Star*, the banner headline was the same size and breadth as the one used months earlier for the story of the actual Crash. The round-up had taken place on a Thursday, the day the *Financial Post* hit the streets, and one cannot resist speculating whether the authorities may have moved when they did to spite Chalmers, knowing that this thorn in their side would suffer the embarrassment of being out of date on its own story for an entire seven days. There was a touch of sheepishness in the *Post*'s comment the following week: "Certain recent arrests are likely to do much to clean up the situation. But these people deserve a fair trial and it's to be hoped that every arrested broker will have a trial that is fair not only to himself but to the public."

On the day of the raid, one of the brokerages affected closed its doors in the late morning, while others lingered into the afternoon, their clerks busily reassuring anxious customers who had every reason to be worried even without the arrests. But many others remained open, though the mood was bleak on Bay, Richmond, and Wellington streets, and in the Bank of Hamilton building near by, where many of the exchange members had suites. A joke began circulating to the effect that meetings in these people's boardrooms commenced with a prayer and ended with an investigation. It was necessary, however, to maintain a more confident front for the public. "We are doing business just as usual," one exchange official commented. "Arrests may come and arrests may go but the mining exchange goes on forever."

But it was not to be. The provincial government *had* been closing in on questionable practices, as the passage of the 1928 security fraud bill indicated. The role of the *Post* was to prod the government by means of a loud and uncharacteristic display, whipping up complaints from small investors and forcing the hand of the other provinces as well. The government reacted in a dramatic and sensational manner because it had been put up to it by the dramatic and sensational stories in the *Post*. Everyone seemed pleased with the results. The premier, Smilin' Howard Ferguson, precipitated no more headline-grabbing arrests but continued to work on the problem, more quietly, as the Depression worsened. In 1934, when the *Securities Exchange Act* was passed in the United States, his successors had wide support in forcing the merger of the Standard into the

TSE. This squeezed out the charlatans and financial bounders, but not before one final epidemic of swindling. This last blaze of glory for the Standard was based on a new gold boom that, ironically, proved a small lifesaver to Canadians still smarting from similar speculations only a few years before.

As part of the plan of action by which he put a moratorium on banking, Franklin Roosevelt, when he came to office in 1933, also ordered an embargo on gold exports. The price of gold rose steadily, setting off another incredible boom in Canada, as worthless old properties were opened once again and wheezing companies, not entirely sound to start with, revitalized. Even after Congress fixed the price at $35 per troy ounce, hope persisted that the price would continue rising, and this too fed the boom. The Standard was closed only after it became obvious this was false expectation. The U.S. government forced still more fast operators to slip across the border. Soon Ontario was again alive with boiler-rooms and bucket shops, as small speculators financed a further scouring of the northland. Between 1932 and 1934 the shares of Dome went from $9 to $32, of Hollinger from $4.25 to $21.25, and of Hudson's Bay from 90 cents to $15.

But the true benefit was felt in the blighted West, even though Ontario and Quebec got the thrust of the boom. Manitoba was especially relieved. Winnipeggers, wrote James H. Gray in *The Winter Years*, "saw it as the economic panacea—the diversifier that would at last rescue western Canada from the tyranny of King Wheat and the one-crop economy. The Manitoba discoveries could not match the big finds in Northern Ontario. But nobody on Portage Avenue would concede any such thing in 1934....The money supplied by the long-shot gamblers in penny shares got a tremendous development going. All across the north country from Bridge River to Flin Flon, to Rice Lake, to Red Lake, to Pickle Lake, to Little Long Lac, to Larder Lake, new communities bloomed around mines in the bush, and jobs created in Vancouver, Winnipeg, Fort William, Sudbury, and Toronto." But even this was almost laughably too little in what by then had become such desperate times.

4

Stock Market Fever

This is getting ahead of the story, however. The story is that of the steep but occasionally jerky rise in market activity leading up to September 1929. A graph could easily show the tall curve. But some device more on the order of an oscilloscope is needed to reveal the electric current then running through the financial community. New highs were being set week after week until, in time, the fantastic lost its appeal as novelty.

The upward trend had begun going crazy in 1927, when prices and volume simply rose and rose throughout the year as though tied somehow to the cumulative effect of the passing seasons. The speculative disease led to one or two outlandish occurrences which few people, trapped in their own context, thought unusual. When prices began slacking off in January 1928, for example, both President Calvin Coolidge and his treasury secretary, Andrew Mellon, spoke out in bold optimism with the deliberate intention of stopping the slide. Later Coolidge made a still more remarkable statement to the effect that he did not consider the amount of brokers' loans too large. Such tactics worked for a time, though it was becoming clear from an array of vital signs—employment, steel production, car-loadings, and the like—that the economy was winding down on both sides of the border.

In the first few months of 1929 the stock markets were restive. The founder of the Federal Reserve System, Paul M. Warburg (after whom would be named the Harvard chair of economics that Galbraith occupied), warned against the "unrestrained speculation" and was hooted down. Moody's Investors Service in New York spoke of the need for market "readjustment". This word would rapidly become popular as the financial world grew polarized, with qualified optimists in one camp and outright bulls in the other. It enabled the user to sound pragmatic without lapsing into cries of woe; it bespoke the belief (not borne out in reality) that the market, though manic-depressive, was still in control. The Harvard Economic Society and other bodies and organizations held to this view as well, in opposition to the outright gloom merchants, who were beginning to find followers of their own. Yet all such people combined were a distinct minority. And the unpredictableness, in any case, promised good as well as bad. The same week Moody's and the Harvard group made their statements prices turned up markedly, beginning a spiral that (allowing for a few faint spells) would continue through the autumn of 1929. In retrospect this was the beginning of the final glide path which ended up in the terrible crash landing.

Floyd Chalmers again:

> I remember one fellow—he's still around but I don't know whether he's got his money any more. He was down in New York and had cottoned onto one of the investment trusts and had bought a lot of shares in companies above their real value, something about $50 million good for $100 million. Anyway, he had $325,000 profit on that. I asked him the obvious question, "Have you actually taken your profit?" "No," he said, "it's going to double." He was going to be a millionaire. Then came the collapse and he was wiped out totally. I think he was paying off his debts for years. There must have been thousands of tragedies of just that kind.

Events in Canada were like a shadow of those in the United States at this time so far as the markets were concerned. One day in November 1928, for instance, trading on the New York Stock Exchange reached almost 7 million shares, a record; Montreal and Toronto reacted in kind, proportionately. The same puppet response could be noted the following months, when the New York exchange suffered its first serious break, with RCA down 72 points, International Harvester down 61½, and Monkey Ward down 29, to name just three prominent examples. But then as now, and in both nations, it was a moot point whether the market's most amazing quality was volatility or resiliency. In February 1929 there was another decline in prices, though less dramatic than the first, and the Federal Reserve began discouraging its member banks from making further loans for the purpose of market speculation.

In March 1929 yet another slip was recorded, with over 8 million shares sold on one day at the NYSE. By now these small calamities were becoming part of the game, though this one would have been far more serious had not the American banking giants banded together to reinforce the market. Matters were taking a crazy zigzag course. Conditions were unstable and yet they were marvellous. Mostly they were almost out of control. The undiminished rush of speculators had been driving up the interest rate for call money, the instantly recallable loans made to brokers. The rate jumped from 6 to 8 to 10 per cent and then from 12 to 15 per cent and finally in March went to 20.

Long before this dizzy height was reached, manufacturing companies had discovered that they got a better return on their capital by lending to speculators than they could by going about their manufacturing. By the time of the Crash, U.S. companies had lent $6.6 billion in this manner and the banks about one-third as much. This only did further harm to the economic foundation. But most people's attention was still on the booming market. In the less dour brokerage offices (even in Toronto) the boardmen who chalked changing prices on giant elevated blackboards had been replaced by boardwomen, who were very young and had short skirts and, in the sexist argot of the times, shapely gams.

The market seesawed through April and May but there were no panics, and this comparatively steady period boosted confidence throughout the summer. There was much talk of how one could tell when one was overstaying a bull market. But almost everybody who was already in felt he should stay a bit longer; people still outside saw this as their last chance to get ahead. In August, the automobile millionaire John J. Raskob published an article in the *Ladies' Home Journal* outlining in detail how people with only $15 per week to invest could make themselves $80,000 in 20 years by following through on a simple stock market gambit.

For the past several years, many large companies had been refinancing in order to expand according to the dictates of the general economic boom. Simpsons had put an issue on the market in 1925, for instance, and Canada Cement did the same in 1928. Massey-Harris was an other example, though its plans got lost in the Crash. Now, in the States as well as in Canada, companies were not simply refinancing and merging but splitting their stock for cosmetic reasons alone. The small investor liked dealing in big numbers and preferred owning 10 shares of Dominion Widget worth $100 total to holding 2 shares at $50 each. It was madness. American brokerage houses had maintained about five hundred branch offices around the country in 1919; now the figure was well over two thousand, and growing. Someone estimated that more than one million American citizens had margin accounts totalling 300 million shares worth God knows what. And this at a time when the population of the entire country, children included, was only 123 million. Two months later, *Variety*, the showbiz gazette, would run its famous headline about Wall Street laying an egg. But right now everyone was bidding the Street break a leg.... Then came September and the beginning of the end.

Once the Crash was history many investors and speculators would confess openly that they had seen it coming and had liquidated at the right moment, with their fortunes more or less intact. At the very least one could find people who claimed to have had foresight enough to continue their gambling on a cash-only basis. A few such people would appear to have been telling the truth, but only a precious few surely.

Mackenzie Williams, a broker with A. E. Ames of Toronto, is one example; he got out in September after the first serious trouble. Among the famous there was Charlie Chaplin, arguably the wealthiest actor in Hollywood at the time. He once told Alistair Cooke that he had pulled out early and transferred his assets to Canada and South Africa, with good results. Cooke has reported no more of the conversation, but Chaplin probably put his money into legitimate gold-mining ventures in the two countries. By that method he could have done very well, as gold proved to be just as attractive in the deflationary times to come as it always has been in inflationary ones, its worth remaining steady while the value of the dollar increased. And then there is the story of Joe Kennedy, the financier and eventual patriarch of the Kennedy clan. Legend has it he ceased being a bull when, riding in an elevator, he overheard the office boys discussing the stock market in some detail. Documented instances of such prescience are scarce, however. Looking back at the period it would almost seem as though there were more prophets of doom forecasting the Crash than people heeding their advice.

Quite a few sets of ears pricked up in late 1928, for example, when Alexander Dana Noyes of the *New York Times* began warning that a severe decline, perhaps even a full-fledged collapse, was imminent. Noyes was the premier financial reporter of the day and is now looked upon as the first giant figure in what is still all too often considered a journalistic backwater. His prediction met with at least some consideration because he was excellent at his job and was scrupulously honest in an age when business reporters were often on the take. What's more, he had foreseen the coming bull market as early as 1923.

In Canada as in the States, the message was coming through. George Gooderham, the Toronto distiller and financial power, was one who spoke publicly about the danger. Another was Sir Charles Gordon, of the Bank of Montreal. And then there was the Bank of Nova Scotia. As early as September 1927 it had sent a confidential memo to its domestic branch managers warning that the level of speculation was becoming too high. It followed this with another report in May 1928. In the intervening months, the document stated, "values on the whole have continued to rise, and so widespread has speculation become that to-day we have an unhealthy, if not dangerous, situation confronting us." Now a third directive, in March 1929, urged managers to scrutinize very carefully any stocks offered as collateral lest it become "necessary for this office to issue definite instructions in regard to stagnant loans."

In fact, by the time of their 1929 annual meetings most of the large chartered banks were actually going on record through the medium of the president's address. Their alarums were out of character, but the public regarded them as the statements of old fuss-budgets, if in fact they paid much attention at all. The Bank of Montreal, say, has paid a dividend on its common stock uninterruptedly since 1828 but it's done so by being conservative to the point of asphyxiation, completely out of step with the vigorous times: this at least was the general feeling among speculators, who took their cues from other quarters.

But the most remarkable reaction was that to a speech by Roger W. Babson, the investment counsellor and publisher of statistical reports. Babson had made his fortune advocating a somewhat dubious "action-reaction" theory of market activity which he claimed was derived from the thoughts of Sir Isaac Newton. For a complex tangle of reasons this well-known doom-sayer created turmoil when, in the first week of September, he cried wolf not only once too often but too well. The result was the first serious break since the Canadian Marconi incident and one with ominous consequences. After that, and for a while at least, new issues continued to appear; volume ran about 4.5 million shares in New York; brokers paid 9 per cent interest on call money and commercial paper went out at 6.5. But thenceforth the optimism was gone and it was optimism (in the garb of greed and credit) that held the whole system together.

A word might be said here about Babson, perhaps the most eccentric figure in the unorthodox financial world of the time. He was an umpteenth-generation New Englander, born in 1875, when the region was still the centre of American cultural life and also the birthplace of intellectual trends the way California is today. Babson resembled many of the famous and obscure faddists of the nineteenth century (the Owenites and other communalists, the Single Taxers, the anti-vivisectionists, and those who built octagonal houses at the urging of Orson Fowler, the phrenologist). But with Babson there was one important difference: he was a crackpot of the right instead of the left.

Although he had been trained in civil engineering, this knowledge found only partial expression in one of his early jobs, which was wiring doorbells for the residents of Gloucester, Massachusetts. His career really began just before the turn of the century when he worked in investment banking in Boston. It was then he got the idea for his *Babson's Reports*, though until these market letters caught on he sold railway stocks which he later admitted were a bit shady. It was also during this period that he contracted tuberculosis. He was cured but the experience made him a health crank, one with unique ideas about hygiene as well as about business. He seems to have invented both the modern paper-towel dispenser and the employee suggestion box, for instance. He believed that windows should be open year round. As a result, his secretaries often had to wear their coats and hats and type with mittens on, using little hammers to strike the keys.

In later years, as the empire grew, Babson branched out into promoting world government and set up an institute for the study of gravity. The two causes were somehow connected in his mind.

"World peace will come only as the Spirit of Jesus grows in the hearts of man and as the principles of birth control are taught to overcrowded nations and the latent power of gravity is used as freely as air, water and sunlight." The quotation is from one of his books. Over the years he wrote about 50—all of them on paper save one which was carved in stone. Babson wore a T-shaped moustache-and-goatee combination. In time it turned to white, giving him an eerie resemblance to the present day Colonel Sanders. That such a person should have influenced the market is bizarre even in the context of that curious month, September 1929.

Tuesday, September 3, would be the first business day after the long Labour Day weekend. For workers this was a respite enforced by law, but New York's sanitation crews were getting extra pay cleaning up after the professional classes. The *Graf Zeppelin* had visited the city, and New York had responded to the occasion (as it did to all such occasions) by staging a ticker-tape parade. On a normal business day, the financial district then went through 4.5 million feet of tape. Now a stripe up the middle of Manhattan was littered with incalculable additional miles of the stuff, thrown out of office windows along with confetti, shredded waste-paper, and whatever else was handy. The celebration had seemed a bit forced, however. At least it did not touch the average middle-class burgher like the news on that Tuesday, when stock prices reached the highest levels they had *ever* achieved in what turned out to be the market's absolute summit—and hence, its turning-point.

In New York even more than Montreal and Toronto, the big advances during the recent months of bullish activity had been in the blue-chip stocks, and September 3 was the final reconfirmation that these were where money could be made. The only comparable across-the-board rises had been the previous March. But the new tallies made the March ones pale. To make the comparisons fairly one must allow for the fact that many of the stocks had split during this six-month period, as prominent stocks in those days always seemed to do.

American Telephone and Telegraph, for instance, had opened on March 3 at 179½ but now peaked at an adjusted price of 335⅝. With General Electric, the figures were 128¾ as against the September 3rd high of 396¼ (adjusted). With Woolworth, the six-month difference was between 180¾ and the adjusted high of 251.

Clearly this was a bonanza time for those holding the choice American industrial and retail stocks, which tended to occupy the attention of a great many small Canadian investors of the more cautious type. On the Montreal Stock Exchange advances were generally less pronounced and not so centred in one area. Steel Company of Canada, Famous Players, Canadian Canners, and various others had flourishes, but the best advances were in the resource industries, with such stocks as International Nickel and Noranda. Oil was especially strong, with both British American and Imperial setting records. On the Standard, however, activity was generally soft despite the release that day of a Dominion Bureau of Statistics report showing 1929 the best year ever in mineral production.

It was in short a very, very good day. If Canadian stocks did not reach quite the heights of the best American ones, there were still more similarities than differences. In both countries, for instance, there was a sense that the highs and the voluminous trading for the day would set the tone for the remainder of the year, now that the drowsy summer was officially past. But there was also shared uncertainty and confusion about the direction of the economy in general and the markets in particular. Perhaps the Montreal *Gazette*'s business page summed up the situation best:

> There is a rather evident sense that we are living under conditions which make reference as to the next turn of events exceptionally difficult. Three different attitudes seem to be taken in regard to the financial future. One is that we have now discovered positively the existence of a new financial and industrial era, in which old rules are wholly abrogated and past experience has no lessons worth considering. Another is that the

recent trend of affairs in industry and in the speculative market cannot last; that its reversal, when it comes, may be severe in proportion to the violence of the movement which is interrupted, but that no one can fix the time and circumstances for the change. The third position, probably occupied by the greater part of the financial community, is that reasoned judgement has been suspended for the present and that, whatever underlying convictions may be entertained, it is just as well to go with the stream while watching the longer horizon carefully.

As the *Gazette* suggested, most people seemed to follow the third course of action. While they did so the second snuck up on them. On Wednesday the fourth the story was the same in both countries. The markets opened with a flurry of activity, with gains outnumbering declines. By noon the lists had generally turned downward, though no one seemed seriously concerned: there was no reason to be.

The following day, September 5, the wire services carried a report of an address Babson made to a national business conference. Babson had predicted a stock market crash that would rival the collapse of the Florida land boom, that mammoth pyramiding of vacation real estate that had caved in after two hurricanes in 1925 and nearly wrecked the state's economy. Babson was quoted as saying that "more people are borrowing and speculating today than ever before in our history. Sooner or later there is a crash coming and it may be a terrific one."

Babson was especially concerned with the recent bluechip market: while more than 600 of the 1,200 issues listed on the NYSE had declined in value since January, the 40 stocks he considered the leaders had gained an average of 80 points, or 42 per cent. He foresaw a corresponding decline of from 60 to 80 points in the Dow Jones average when the collapse came. There were also rumours that day (groundless, as it happened) that the Bank of England was about to change its discount rate, forcing the Fed to follow suit. But most of the reaction arose from the fact that reports of Babson's speech were included on the ticker.

What happened next was more important than dramatic. There was no wholesale withdrawal by all types of investors as there would be later. Nor were there even individual days disastrous enough to be distinguished with the prefix "black", as there would be in October. Rather, the logic of Babson's remarks began to sink in, giving many medium-sized gold diggers the reason they needed for unloading. Prices were consistently erratic. On the fifth, Wall Street trading jerked forward while the MSE generally declined, the TSE slowed down less willingly, and the mining exchange showed a slight improvement. At least conditions in Canada could be ascribed to a new tightness of money arising from moves on the part of the banks and withdrawal from the call money market by the Dominion's larger companies. It took another day for the New York crisis to build momentum and for its shock waves to reach Canada.

Late Friday the front page of the *Calgary Herald* was typical with the headline "STOCK MARKET SCARE". The Montreal *Gazette* was more detailed, indicating how small speculators had been wiped out in the last hour of trading in New York. "Statement by Babson and Increase in Brokers' Loans Main Causes of Break" ran a subhead.

The big money men on Wall Street were taken aback. They couldn't comprehend how a Babson speech, bald as it was, could have triggered such a reaction. After all, Babson had a reputation as a "calamity howler", and the community was quick to say it never paid that much attention to him in the past. "Regardless of the accuracy of his prediction," the *Mail and Empire* stated, "the statement had a bearish influence." It succeeded in spooking just enough people to throw a spanner in the (by this time) very precarious brokers' loan situation.

The trouble had come in the last hour of trading on Wall Street. But since the ticker was running an hour behind, as it often was in the 1920s when the market fluctuated wildly, the news didn't come out until after the trading floors had closed. This made for a mood of anxiety overnight in Montreal and Toronto, where reverses in New York were usually reflected fully even though American gains often had little corresponding effect.

The next morning was to be an important one for both countries, though in Canada it was more nervous than action filled. When the wires opened, New York brokers began sending out responses to Babson. Investors should not allow themselves to be stampeded, they said, by a mere statistician. Anyway, there were plenty of other statisticians and economists who did not share Babson's prognosis.

But the damage had been done. In New York, more than a billion dollars in share value was lost when reality had its way with the largely inflated prices on the Big Board. In Canada there were no breaks so serious, though the situation was certainly edgy, and with some analogous occurrences. No single group of stocks stood up well; this was most obvious in the case of oils, which had lately been buoyant. Yet British American was perky amid rumours of a stock split; and CPR was strong despite the fact rails were doing badly in the States.

Not that there wasn't excitement here. The stock of Teck-Hughes dropped to nearly five dollars. According to the *Daily Star*, "Panicky talk was heard in the board rooms of many Toronto brokerage houses.... This was a drop of approximately $6 million in market value over the weekend, and the air was so filled with rumours that scarcely anyone was willing to believe anything good about this famous gold mine, which only a short time ago was the favourite of the Street."

It had been a shortened week but the four days had been packed with confusion and fear. Now the Saturday papers tried to assess the situation calmly. To be sure, Canadian investors on balance had not been upset by Babson's remarks in quite the same way the Americans had. But neither was Canada so resilient as the States. In the break of the preceding March we had not taken quite so severe a beating, but then we had recovered far more slowly than New York. And it seemed as though this pattern was about to repeat itself here, and for fairly obvious reasons.

American prosperity was still blatant; in Canada, the economy was perhaps slowing down a bit more obviously, as exemplified by the disordered wheat situation. Also, the spirit of optimism in the States had always seemed more fluid. There was, however, a certain Canadian belief in the status quo that helped keep us going. "The entire action of the markets in the past few days," according to the *Gazette*, "lends colour to the theory held in important circles that no change in the main trend is imminent [though] technical readjustments [will be] quite logical developments from time to time." But no. Some stocks actually surpassed the highs of September 3, though the market basically proceeded in a sideways crawl, up a bit here, then down, then up but less than previously. The trend was generally downward from this point on and matters were never quite the same.

5

Life and Death
of the Grain Exchange

The Winnipeg Grain Exchange still stands on Lombard Street, one giant block from Portage and Main, but the atmosphere inside will never again be what it was in the 1920s. In 1935 Mackenzie King reintroduced the Canadian Wheat Board and later made it the sole marketing agent of what formerly had been bought and sold by private companies and daring individuals. The exchange is now permitted to trade only in coarse grains such as flax, barley, rye, and oats, and the offices along its splendid old corridors are filled mainly with not very interesting commodities brokers. Besides, the spirit which made the exchange one of the most exciting places in Canada passed forever from the psychological landscape after the steady deterioration of the grain market in the early 1930s.

Hopeful gold diggers were just as prevalent on the Prairies as they were elsewhere but tended to speculate in grain (and also, to some extent, in oil) rather than in securities listed on the eastern stock exchanges. So widespread and haphazard was their gambling, and so small the capital needed to begin, that the 10-storey building on Lombard could better be compared with the Standard mining exchange in Toronto. The difference, as John Kenneth

Galbraith points out, is that "the Toronto mining exchange bore more relation to Woodbine race track than to anything going on in the economy." In grain, by contrast, the outside economy was crucial. The collapse, when it came, was caused not so much by the weight of speculation, tremendous though it was, as by political developments in other parts of the world. This was no consolation to the people involved, of course, especially after Nature turned against them. But the wheat market was at best unstable long before the dust bowls concentrated everyone's attention.

It's difficult for most people today to cast themselves back to how it must have been when Canada was not yet so urban a country. Figures for 1931, for instance, showed 29 per cent of the work force engaged in farming, as against only 15 per cent in the next biggest group, manufacturing. The CPR continued to run a few colonization cars, though the basic settlement of the West, founded on wheat and railways, had already been completed. On balance, the entire region was in a prosperous state that periodically verged on boom, though there had been the great recession immediately after the First World War. It would become clear, in fact, that the war years were a kind of dividing line: whether times afterward were good or bad, they would not be good or bad in quite the same ways.

Prior to the war, many saw the brightest future for the West in cattle. Farming played a bigger role than ranching; arable land is what had brought the immigrants. Acreage was growing significantly year by year and there were periodical high spots, as in 1901 when the crop was so large as to occasion a severe shortage of rolling stock. But the cities were being built by the cattle aristocracy typified by Sir James Lougheed; they were the movers and shakers, at least for a time. The western provinces were growing so fast (Manitoba went from 150,000 people in 1891 to almost half a million 20 years later) that the ranchers couldn't keep up with demand. By 1911, for instance, cattle shipped from Ontario were making up a good deal of the Winnipeg market. Then the Americans began restricting the importation of Canadian cattle after

Argentina, on the world scene, undersold Canada on the market for chilled beef. By the time the war began, wheat was the established beneficiary of geopolitical and economic momentum.

In 1915, the crop for the first time exceeded 300 million bushels, as opposed to 150 or 200 million in the preceding couple of years, which had themselves set impressive records. The jump in the amount of land under cultivation (almost 14 million acres) had coupled with good weather and a minimum of pestilence to do what had seemed blatantly impossible only a few years earlier. The farmers were in the chips. As farmers with cash in their pockets have done ever since, they put money into equipment, only to find later that the cost of carrying the rest on credit was more than they could handle.

For sure enough the bonanza was short-lived. The following year wheat stem rust badly hurt the crop in Manitoba and various other circumstances conspired against those in Saskatchewan and Alberta. The downward trend persisted through 1918 and 1919, the worst years for Prairie farmers in two decades. Yet the price for grain was high because of the war in Europe, with the Allies buying all they could. In 1917, in fact, the federal government set up the Canadian Wheat Board as an emergency measure to provide the war effort with as much grain as possible. It was reinstated briefly in 1919 and again in 1921. By that time another force, the wheat pools, was about to enter the equation.

Creation of the Wheat Board is perhaps what first gave rise to the old saying that wheat is 13 per cent protein and 87 per cent politics. The grievances of the farming community, however, predated the board's establishment by a couple of generations. As always, transportation was the major headache. Even before the CPR was completed in 1885, there were complaints about the monopoly it enjoyed. Then, as now, there was unending tension about rates, and most particularly the 1897 Crowsnest Pass Agreement whereby the government funded many branch lines in return for the lower fare on grain bound for port. Most persistent of all, however, were complaints about the private elevator companies. Farmers took it as common knowledge that when they trucked their wheat to the elevators for payment in cash they would be cheated on the grading system and perhaps also on the volume by weight. There were royal commissions from time to time, but years passed before they took marketing into their own hands.

Prairie farmers had long been experimenting with the sort of elemental agrarian socialism from which so much of Canadian radicalism springs. While some of the recent immigrants were trying to transplant certain principles of communalism, not often with much success, those better established made great headway adapting the co-operative movement to their own needs. What could not be grown or made had to be bought, and a co-op existed for the bulk purchase of almost every farm staple—one for coal oil, for instance, and another for barbed wire. There were even long-established co-operatively owned elevators. There was, however, no such system for the actual marketing of wheat until Aaron Sapiro arrived on the scene in 1923.

Sapiro had begun life as a street kid in Oakland, California, and was now a San Francisco lawyer with a self-assigned mission to organize the North American farmer along lines of self-help, self-determination, and mass cooperation. This would lead in time to an infamous legal battle with Henry Ford, who in one of his frequent crackpot outpourings accused Sapiro of participating in an international Jewish conspiracy to control the world's food supply. But long before his libel action Sapiro came to the notice of the Calgary *Herald*. Whether from altruism or enterprise or some combination of the two, the *Herald* brought Sapiro to Alberta, where he made appeals to the farmers' instinct for self-preservation and mesmerized them with his oratorical style. The result was the Alberta Wheat Pool begun that year. Sapiro then moved on and organized the Saskatchewan Wheat Pool in 1924 and Manitoba Pool Elevators in 1925.

The pools were intended to level out the incessant rising and dipping of wheat prices caused by speculation on the Winnipeg exchange. Such volatility made life so unpredictable for the farmer that on occasion he would have no profit even on a good crop. But the pools did not immediately have this desired effect for one simple reason: the farmers were inveterate small-time gamblers. Like their colleagues on the Standard in Toronto, the exchange members met critics with a pat answer which was not quite logical. The advantage of the exchange, they held, was that it brought together a great mass of speculators who themselves took the beating when prices dropped, sparing the farmers the hardest blows. The difficulty with this syllogism was that the speculators and the farmers were very often one and the same. The wheat-growers who belonged to the pools and took such pride in their group effort at orderly marketing were addicted to decadent individualism.

Taking flyers on the market is what they did instead of gambling in stocks, those who were caught up in the spirit of the times. When I. W. C. Solloway of Solloway, Mills and Company began opening western branches of his bucket-shop enterprise he found he had to add wheat departments. These soon became one of the most profitable parts of his operation. When he would make his regular visits to Calgary and invite his clients up for a drink in his suite in the Palliser Hotel, it seemed as though half of the city was there. And this was Calgary, where the locals usually eschewed Toronto mining stocks for Vancouver ones and for western oil ventures. Their presence was a boozy testament to the grip of wheat fever.

Like the one in Calgary, the Winnipeg exchange had been built in 1909. Its appearance betrayed a time, only a generation earlier, when brass and hardwoods had been used freely, in grain exchanges no less than in saloons, to compensate for the proximity of the frontier in time and distance. A 1920 expansion program made it for a while the largest office building in the Empire. It had a smoking-room with cuspidors and also a billiard room. The latter included some slot machines, at least until a book-keeper employed in one of the brokerages tried to hit the jackpot with four thousand dollars in change he had embezzled from the firm.

By the 1920s, the exchange was the hub of what, for the time, was a very sophisticated communications network. On the sixth floor were the pits, two octagonal areas resembling old-fashioned operating theatres. One was for wheat, the other exclusively for the coarse grains that accounted for about 10 per cent of the trading. Orders men and brokers milled about the trading floor while boardmen paced a 100-foot catwalk. Prices and relevant data were displayed instantaneously as received from the floor. So was news of the New York, Chicago, Liverpool, Minneapolis, and Duluth exchanges. A complicated series of telegraph link-ups was kept busy, as were banks of telephones.

Winnipeg was the centre of all such activity across the West, and grain company reps at the remotest elevator acted as unofficial brokers and messengers, sending and passing along to locals the latest prices and information. Those who owned them strained at the headpieces of their primitive old crystal sets to get the same information from the few widely spaced commercial radio stations. Farmers everywhere west of the Lakehead seemed to go about their work with one ear cocked for the news from the exchange.

These were not, it should be noted, sophisticated commodities speculators like many of today's farmers, with subscriptions to the *Financial Post* and Reuters wire machines in their homes. They did not deal in futures as insurance against poor crops and bad years but gambled for the sheer neurosis of doing so, like the most advanced lottery addicts of today.

In Chicago, the grain exchange was a big and sometimes bloodthirsty business. Men such as Arthur W. Cutten would deal in millions of bushels at a time and in the case of some thinly traded commodities, such as May oats, succeed in cornering the market and fixing the price almost at will. Their favourite scheme was to buy October futures and sell May futures, purchasing wheat far out in the boondocks with the intention of selling in Chicago at an added profit. In time, such grain men, along with some made suddenly wealthy by the boom in automobiles, would stage a midwestern invasion of Wall Street. But on the Winnipeg exchange matters were different. The volume was smaller, and most of it derived from individual farmers and hangers-on, eager for a quick turnover, a fast buck. Estimates have placed the number of successful speculators at only 1 in 20, and even then success was fleeting and came in all sizes, most of them small.

The exchange was without doubt an important part of the international food-marketing apparatus. It reacted quickly to developments in Europe and Latin America, say, and the sensitivity was mutual. Its members included elevator companies, terminal companies, millers, exporters, and Great Lakes fleets, as well as a certain number of American corporate giants and international trading concerns. But there were also blocs of options brokers, catering to the individual gambler. Except during the summer bull markets, when the professional classes joined in, their customers were usually farmers. Those in Manitoba would frequently make excuses to journey to Winnipeg for periods of up to a month with the sole purpose of joining the fray. They would put up at some drovers' hotel perhaps and spend their days in option brokers' offices, each with its own board and an array of tout sheets and other propaganda.

> Anybody with $100 to risk [writes James H. Gray in *The Roar of the Twenties*] could walk into an option broker's office, deposit the $100, and buy 1,000 bushels of wheat futures on a ten-cent margin. For every cent that the price moved upward or downward, the gambler would gain or lose $10. If the price dropped five cents a bushel, the broker might ask him to put up another $50 to maintain his ten-cent margin. If the price rose by ten cents, he could sell out and pocket $100 in profit, less $2.50 commission to the broker. Or, by using his profit as margin he could buy another 1,000 bushels. Then, as the market rose or fell, he would win or lose $20 for every cent of rise and fall.

The natural tendency was to roll over any profit instead of getting out with the cash while the getting was good.

If there was any doubt that the exchange catered to the gamblers, it was abolished each afternoon when, once the trading floor had been swept of litter, the privileges market began. This was the game of puts 'n' calls—in effect, one-day futures contracts that allowed the gambler to bet which way the market would go the following day. It cost only one dollar to join the action. Another peculiarity of the grain exchange as opposed to the stock market was that the activity was highly seasonal; it followed, or was at least related to, the natural cycle of agriculture.

The price of grain was always lower in the autumn than in the spring because autumn was when the farmers sold their harvest to the elevators. That a bull market would prevail in the spring and summer, in anticipation of the harvest and a price rise, was taken for granted. But that being the case, there was less rhyme and reason in the price of grain from autumn to autumn than one would imagine, at least when one disallowed the impact of changing world conditions.

Textbook economists would have it that the price went up when the crop was poor and a scarcity resulted. In theory, it follows that the price must perforce have gone down when a bumper crop created a glut on the market. In actual practice, however, whenever the yield was bad the farmer covered himself by planting more than usual. There was thus a glut even during bad times and this kept the price from rising. Prices would indeed rise when the bullish season approached, however. It was an article of faith that most speculators joined the fray only after the bull trend was already established.

For some months each year, then, the Winnipeg exchange would be relatively quiet and the visitors' gallery bare. At other times, however, commotion would take over, brokers' back shops would work far into the night vainly trying to keep up with the paperwork, and visitors would jam the gallery and spill out into the corridor, only to clamber onto the floor when the market broke. In 1924, however, the bull market got out of whack and continued in that condition through the fall and winter, when the farmers came to town for their annual binge. The result was that the market detached itself from reality, culminating on January 29, 1925. This date didn't exactly mark the collapse of the grain market. But it did prove beyond a doubt the dangerous instability which let the market slide into nothingness once the stock disaster set off its chain reaction.

In 1923 the farmers had had a bumper crop, harvesting 452 million bushels; the average yield on the Prairies as a whole had been over 21 bushels per acre, or the first figure to equal that of 1915. By comparison, 1924 had been only a routine year. The crop looked good in Manitoba but the results in Alberta and Saskatchewan were below normal; total harvest for the three together was only 235 million bushels. By the early fall the price was steady at about $1.35 per bushel for October delivery and $1.30 for delivery the following May. But then bad weather at home and other calamities outside Canada brought people's speculative impulses to the surface.

Trading became so heavy that brokerage employees slept in the building, fully dressed and suffering sore throats, or else took to hotel rooms across the street arranged by their bosses. It looked as though the farmers' worries about the crop would work in tandem with the long-term optimism of the big traders to boost the price to the $2 mark. Although this price had been reached briefly years earlier, it had become again a psychological breaking-point, like the mythical 1,000 for the Dow Jones average. As December became January the price was $1.75. Then, on Friday, January 23, the magic line was crossed. The floor was swarming as it usually did only in summer.

But at least some of the excitement must have been vocal anxiety at what the board would do next. Would the price actually climb above $2 or would it slowly recede? Or would the speculators consider this peak the ultimate and touch off a wave of panic selling? Once again the galleries emptied as the trading floor became a human traffic jam. All across the Prairies others felt the nervous tension vicariously.

As it happened, the market did seem to stall at $2 for a while, but very soon the price had edged up by two cents on the bushel. This set off a fickle delusion that the next plateau would be $2.25, a view that seemed to gain credence when stories circulated about an apparent drought in the Soviet Union. And indeed during the rest of the week the figure did rise to a remarkable $2.20 ⅞ after publicity surrounding the exchange brought hordes of fresh gamblers in off the streets. Then came the 29th, the single most memorable day in the history of western grain speculation.

Reports conflict as to precisely what happened when and, most especially, why. The exchange opened that morning with May wheat at $2.20. The crowd was perhaps even larger than it had been during the past few days. There was a buy! buy! buy! atmosphere like the jump! jump! jump! one associates with ugly sidewalk crowds watching a potential suicide on a high ledge. And then in the span of a quarter-hour the price had fallen to $2.10. "I was there at the time, running in and out of the trading floor," says James Gray. "You could have heard the excitement for blocks away if the windows had been open, as they were in the summertime. There was a tumult that just shook the building." Some person—whose name, if it were ever known, has now been lost to history—had done it, yelled fire in the crowded theatre and sent everyone running for the exits. The pace was frantic. The price of wheat made a series of minute gains and took equally small losses until at closing time the figure stood at $2.14.

Saturday was another teeter-totter but by Monday it became clear that the general trend was to be rapidly down. A great number of speculators, like guests who didn't know when the party was over, refused to pull out even after the price sank back to its pre-$2 levels, and most of these were finally cut down in early February when the price fell 7½ cents in one day. That was the last belated spasm. Once it was over, prices firmed up again, but only as though in long preparation for the further disasters of 1928 and afterward. Typically for the grain market, these later disasters began in good fortune and amid rejoicing.

The wheat crop of 1928 was the biggest ever on the Prairies—more than 544 million bushels. This was the first time the figure had passed the 500-million mark. One gets some sense of its magnitude if one considers that, despite the increased acreage and better technology of later years, the 600-million point was not to be passed until 1952. But though the 1928 harvest was indeed remarkable, it was of a poor quality because of an unconscionably early frost. It was far below that of our old competitor Argentina. Having insufficient storage facilities, Argentina had to flood the world market, an action which naturally pulled the price down. The Argentine wheat in fact sold for as much as 20 cents less than Canadian, which cost Canada some of its best customers, such as the giant British mills. The wheat pools had no choice but to borrow enormous sums from the banks and store as much of the grain as possible with the hope that the market would be better in 1929. But that hope was misplaced.

The quality of the 1929 harvest was better but the yield was only half that of the previous year and 66 per cent of the decade's average; combined with the 1928 surplus, however, it would still have made a decent showing. For a time, in fact, the picture was rosy, at least for Canadians. By the spring of 1929 the first dust bowls had struck the United States and by summer there was imminent danger of another international shortage, which would have left the wheat pools in a pretty position. The price rose and fell in accord with those waves of expectation. Then came dramatic reverses in the total world situation. Italy and Germany had good crops and this kept Britain from returning to Canadian suppliers, and France actually became a wheat-exporting nation for the first time. There were even rumours, which most everybody believed, that the United States would soon have a national wheat pool run by the federal government. Then came the Wall Street crash.

Just as the Crash did not cause the Depression, neither did it cause the bottom to fall out of the wheat market. But the stock market fiasco was the last and deadliest blow to the one-crop economy. As late as August 1929 wheat on the Winnipeg exchange was still trading (on a good day) above the one-dollar-a-bushel level. But the high for the month of October was only 78 cents, the low 69½. Reaction to the Crash was swift around the world as the industrial countries quickly erected tariff barriers and scrambled to defend the economic high ground. Then as one country after another moved to keep out wheat imports, a little string of other misfortunes befell the market. In 1930, the Russians turned out to have had a good surplus and re-entered the export field. Even India registered a big oversupply. And as the competition increased, the markets shrank. The price of silver went all to hell and this meant that China, then in the middle of a civil war, was unable to take wheat off Canada's hands. The eastern bankers began closing in on the pools and the farmers, demanding repayment of money lent in 1928.

The pools were forced to tighten up, and on November 18 this caused another off-season crash on the exchange, with the price falling 8⅜ cents from the previous day's close to a mere 55 cents a bushel. Later on the situation got even worse, for by this time the weather had joined the fray: droughts, dust bowls, grasshopper plagues, and thousands of farms, indeed whole sections of provinces, abandoned, and people living on relief scrip.

Memoirs of the Depression in the West abound; they've become in fact part of the country's living folklore. One person with a story of special ironic relevance to the grain situation is Richard S. Malone, the former publisher of the *Globe and Mail*. During the worst days of the Depression he was struggling to keep afloat the Regina *Leader Post*, from whose office, at noon, it was sometimes impossible to see across Hamilton Street, so fiercely was the dust blowing.

At one time the subscription price for the paper was down to ten cents a week. Even at that the salesmen didn't get cash direct. They'd go out into the country and take chickens in exchange for a subscription. The rate was five or six chickens to the dollar. The salesmen would take the chickens to the packing house and get a receipt, which would be recognized by the Audit Bureau of Circulations as official proof of a bona fide subscriber. In Alberta they tried to get wheat recognized by the ABC, but the price went so low, around forty cents a bushel, that it wasn't worth the price of the newspaper.

Only a few years before, $10 million at a time had been riding on wheat at the Winnipeg Grain Exchange. Now it was almost literally impossible to give the stuff away. At least when the stock markets came unstuck it provided an opportunity for many shrewd speculators (Gordon Sinclair is perhaps the most famous Canadian example) to begin hoarding securities at bargain prices. But with wheat, the system didn't work that way. The ruined were ruined with no immediate prospect of recovery. As late as the approach of the Second World War, the Prairies were full of land no one could reclaim and the building on Lombard Street was full of broken men on wooden benches who had been high rollers in the 1920s.

6

King Cutten

During the 1930s two of Chicago's most famous adopted sons were charged with income tax evasion on a grand scale. One of the accused was Al Capone. The other, in an unrelated case, was Arthur W. Cutten, a Canadian. Cutten's name has not survived the passage of time the way Capone's has, even though Cutten was by far the more mysterious figure and was, according to the present-day economic historian Robert Sobel, "as famous on Wall Street as Babe Ruth and Ty Cobb were in baseball". It has scarcely survived at all in fact, which is curious considering the pattern of his career.

Cutten went from being a folk hero in Canada, looked up to as one of the great tycoons of the age, to being a pariah all over North America, despised for the large role he had played in the Crash. Financially, his is one of the biggest success stories of Canadian and American business history but in public-relations terms one of the greatest failures. Cutten was among a handful of powerful men who seemed to be manipulating the prices of certain key stocks in 1929, thus accelerating the boom and hastening the bust. But he did not suffer as ordinary people did when the end came. Stories at the time about his switching from bull to bear and making a further fortune on everyone else's misery are not exactly true. There is no mistaking, however, that Cutten came out ahead. No one who knew him, or knew about him, would have expected any less.

Nowadays when Cutten is remembered at all, which is seldom, it is as the man who helped rig Wall Street. But such was not the case in the late 1920s. Cutten was viewed with awe by a generation that still admired the robber-baron spirit and took Horatio Alger pluckiness seriously. It was an age when successful businessmen were everyday gods and cleverness was as fashionable a quality in commerce as in popular music. Certainly this was very much the case in the States, where young *Time* magazine's 1929 man of the year was Walter P. Chrysler. Here was a fellow who had started out as a five-cents-an-hour railway workshop apprentice and whose education consisted of a correspondence course—but who was now the leading comer among automobile magnates. His story was a romantic counterweight to the dreary side of business, another redundant justification of money-making and a further proof that the new corporate spirit was not necessarily at odds with individualism.

In Canada the same attitude prevailed but it was mixed with a great respect for the old distinguished elite, such as Sir Herbert Holt. This did not detract, however, from the open admiration for cheeky hustlers like Harry (later Sir Harry) Oakes, whom many people regarded as a lovable character right up until the day of his murder—and all because he had discovered a major gold mine. As an object of public attention, Cutten fell somewhere between these extremes. He was as clever as he was reticent, which was saying a great deal. And since he spent most of his life in the States, he also enjoyed the special benefit of that almost official pride Canadians have in one who hits the big time there while remaining blasé.

Cutten was born in 1870 in Guelph, Ontario. The town would one day rank him as its most important native, after Edward Johnson, "the world's greatest tenor", and James J. Hill, one of the founders of the Canadian Pacific Railway. Hill's example is supposed to have stirred young Cutten into quitting the place, and in

1890 he moved to Chicago, which already had enough businessmen from north of the border to support a monthly magazine called the *Canadian American*. Cutten's first job was as a clerk in Marshall Field's department store but he soon moved over to work as a seven-dollars-a-week office boy and book-keeper with a grain brokerage specializing in corn and wheat. Fourteen years with the firm, he soon rose to the position of trader and learned his business buying commodities on other people's behalf.

Then, in 1906, the year he married a young Chicago woman named Maud Boomer, he decided to become a trader on his own. He scraped together three thousand dollars for a seat on the Chicago Board of Trade, but at first kept the decision to himself. One morning he simply failed to materialize at his desk. Shortly after the market opened for the day, his boss came upon him just inside the trading floor, scribbling furiously on a pad. "What in blazes are you doing in here, Art?" his employer wanted to know.

"Oh, I forgot to tell you," Cutten replied, "I want to be fired. I'm on my own now."

It's no exaggeration to say that from this point on he was one of the nation's most successful speculators. He was also one of the most mysterious and close-mouthed, and altogether contrary to the image of the overfed bellicose capitalist of the Teddy Roosevelt era. Cutten in fact was an undersized man with short-cropped grey hair, a toothbrush moustache, and rimless glasses, and his shyness was extreme. He and his wife seldom entertained at their home on Lake Shore Drive; at the exclusive clubs to which he belonged his presence was only a rumour. And at work he was similarly elusive. In his company's small office in the Board of Trade, a desk was kept clear for him, like a dinner setting for some uncle whose death the family could not cope with. But he seldom showed up, though on the exchange itself his behaviour was a different story.

On the perpetually frantic floor, the one Frank Norris captured in his novel *The Pit*, Cutten was as tough as they come in the endless series of greed tournaments, and bemoaned the absence of worthy contenders. "There are so many wrecks down there in the pit," he told an interviewer. "If I had a son I wouldn't let him touch it with a ten-foot pole. People call themselves brokers, but they are only part of that—the 'broke' part." This was an unusual outburst for someone with so taciturn a public nature. But it gave a pretty good hint of the tenacity that lay beneath the surface. So did a brush with the world of crime.

One of Cutten's major pleasures was his eight-hundred-acre country property in DuPage County, Illinois, 25 miles from downtown Chicago. Owning a spread enabled him to claim special kinship with the farmers, though in fact he was often betting against their success when he went short in the commodities market. The only time he ever listed his occupation officially was when he identified himself before a federal government inquiry as "a cash grain merchant and a dirt farmer". But the lavishness of his place was too well known for this description to deceive anyone but himself, and in 1922 nine gunmen broke into the house, taking cash, jewellery, and rare liquors totalling about fifty thousand dollars. Before leaving they locked Maud, Cutten, and his brother Harry in a vault, where, Cutten said, "we might have suffocated."

Local authorities were unable to solve the case, so Cutten decided to take matters into his own hands. He hired private detectives in numbers entirely out of proportion to the crime. He was also said to have used the influence of Jake Lingle, the Chicago *Tribune* police reporter (later murdered) who was not so secretly in the pay of the Capone interests. The most promising clue was the appearance of some of the exotic liquors from Cutten's collection at a Chicago underworld resort. But the matter dragged on. It took Cutten a decade and cost him a reported $500,000 to bring the nine men to justice. The last one at liberty, Casper Rosenberg, said in exhaustion on surrendering in 1932: "1 can't go on any longer, always hiding. Cutten wins."

Cutten then let the man go, saying, "Send him back where he is building a character for himself." He also helped arrange the parole of another of the nine.

This and lesser stories were told and retold in the LaSalle Street financial district of Chicago and along Portage Avenue in Winnipeg and in other places where commodities mattered, as though through repetition one could get a handle on wily old Cutten, who at one time controlled more grain than any other person in the world. Cutten himself never embellished rumours, although, like Howard Hughes in a later time, when he did break his silence he did so with some style.

In 1922, for instance, he confessed to one transaction that had cost him a mint, but most of his deals were successful in the extreme. In 1924, he bought, for 70 cents a bushel, corn that everyone else assumed would drop in price. But he later sold it at $1.10 and up per bushel, he said, realizing up to 40 cents or so profit per bushel on the last 300,000 units. Fellow traders put his take on that one at $1.5 or $2 million. The story became another favourite of jealous contemporaries, though this was only one of many killings he had made on grain in the past few years. Although Cutten expressed disdain for amateur speculators who cluttered up the market, he once put them next to a good thing. He publicly forecast that wheat, then selling at $1.70 per bushel for delivery in May, would cross $2. The market was flooded. A month later the wheat went for $2.05 and after receding a bit rose up to $2 exactly.

There's no telling how much money Cutten made in Chicago. He was already a millionaire many times over when the big traders came under supervision of the federal government, but even then the figures were not revealed. It is recorded, however, that in one year he paid more income tax that any other individual in Chicago—$540,000, or $100,000 more than the next most notorious operator, old James W. Patten. This was in 1925, the year Chicago ceased being big enough and Cutten branched out into the New York Stock Exchange with his customary mixture of cunning and quiet. Within a year he was one of the strongest forces on Wall Street. He was 54 years old and still liked to refer to himself as a farmer.

It is at this point that the most nagging questions about Cutten began arising, but they are not always questions for which answers exist. What is certain is that, during his first years in the big market, Cutten was a fierce bull who cleared huge profits along with other men of his fiscal stature, though not always in strict partnership with them. He would never confirm that he and his friends made $10 million in 1927 on the stock of Baldwin Locomotive, of which he was a director. Nor would he comment on pretty good rumours that they had made anywhere from $18 to $35 million on Montgomery Ward in 1929. He would later tell the Senate's banking committee, however, that he and his cronies split $12 million in profits from deals in Sinclair Consolidated Oil Companies (Cutten was also a director of both Monkey Ward and Sinclair). One fact, though, is indisputable: he was part of one or more insider consortiums that, in the spring of 1929, did a great deal to boost stock prices higher than they had ever been before.

This was at the time when prices were steadily escalating but the market was at its most volatile, given to unexpected spasms and contractions as one authority after another predicted a collapse, only to be scoffed at by the others. The atmosphere was nervous but mostly with the nervousness one feels when matters are going too well, too fast. The situation became alarming (or alarmingly good) around the week beginning Monday, March 6. General Motors, which had opened at 139¾ the previous Friday, went over 150 by Tuesday; one day GM accounted for one-third of all the shares traded. But within days attention turned instead to the even more dramatic situation of Radio Corporation of America, which gained 12¾ points in one day. United States Steel and that old favourite, Montgomery Ward, were dramatic cases, too. But then it's fitting that there should have been a rise in automobiles and radios, the two devices which had seemed exotic luxuries only a few years before but were now necessities of North American life as the days of prosperity rolled on. There was more than irony at work here, however. Why prices moved as they did was partly because men like

Cutten, with great fortunes to play with, were pumping them up artificially. Many of these were veterans of the auto business.

In addition to Cutten, for instance, the cast included William Crapo Durant, who had put together General Motors in the first place, and John J. Raskob, the GM director who had deposed him and who listed his occupation in *Who's Who* as, simply, "capitalist". Also involved were the Fisher brothers (seven of them), who had sold their Fisher Body plants. Throughout the spring these and perhaps 15 other men transferred more and more of their fortunes into blue chips, counting on the gold-digging instincts of the masses to make them richer. Soon speculators who had been scared off by the fits-and-starts nature of the market spiral were returning en masse. As the spring went on, Radio (as it was then nicknamed) and GM were replaced for a time by other hot stocks. American Telephone and Telegraph, New York Central, Union Carbide, Westinghouse, Woolworth, and a Cutten favourite, Yellow Cab, all had their hour in the sun.

There were sudden slips which took people's breath away for a second, as in June when a twitchy San Francisco Stock Exchange touched off a minor panic across the country. But basically the market continued to climb. In May the Federal Reserve tried to stem the speculation by raising the rediscount rate. After all, lowering it in 1927 is what had helped give the bull market such a big push in the first place. But nothing seemed to work. A great many paper fortunes were being made and lost, but Cutten and his peers were unchallenged masters of the market. Everyone wanted to know them a bit better in order to figure out their methods or at least get a seat on their bandwagon.

At this point Cutten made a curious decision affecting his old home town in Ontario. He had not lived in Canada for almost 30 years, though it was said he sometimes visited siblings in Guelph and Toronto and even contributed, usually anonymously, to local charities. Yet in April he announced his intention of giving the residents of Guelph a $2-million gift in the form of a modern hotel, with a full-size golf course and a general recreation area. It was all to be done in the proper style. The hotel, which would include a ballroom large enough for two thousand people, would be designed by Benjamin Marshall, the architect of the Drake Hotel in Chicago; the CPR agreed to manage it as part of a deal Cutten struck with the railway's president, his friend E. W. Beatty. "Everywhere in Guelph smiles appear at the mention of the name of Arthur Cutten," wrote a Toronto *Mail and Empire* reporter. A bus driver stated proudly how Cutten, the last time he was there, honoured the bus with his presence instead of being chauffeured around town. And many local people were getting stock tips from Cutten, or so they claimed. Now the Cutten name was to be as prominent in Guelph as Lord Beaverbrook's would one day be in Fredericton. This at least was the expectation. John Kenneth Galbraith was at Guelph's Ontario Agricultural College at the time, before moving to Berkeley during the Depression.

In the late 1920s Cutten was one of the vague unspoken heroes of the community. The Ontario government in 1927 had brought G. I. Christie back to head the college there—he had been director of extension at Purdue and United States Department of Agriculture director in the First World War. A strident, disingenuous figure whose positive side was a way of getting things done, which was needed at Guelph at the time. On the other hand [laughs] his vision of scientific and academic achievement was ridiculous. He was what we call here a farm bureau politician. In any event, he began promoting an area between the lake and the campus as a golf course and got Cutten to promise the money. Cutten was around, though those of us there never saw him. But we heard of him as one of the great philanthropic figures of all time, on the level of some great Christian charity. We didn't know how he made all that money.

It is difficult in today's atmosphere to recapture the way the announcement of Cutten's gift excited the little town and the rest of

Ontario. Even Cutten was surprised. "I think everybody is making too much of this," he said. "I happen to have the money, Guelph happens to be my old home, the friends of my early youth are here, and I am willing to give the money, and the old town is willing to take it. So why should there be all this fuss about it? The whole transaction is really a very simple one."

Or was it? When the Crash came, Guelph was reportedly the hardest-hit city of its size in Canada, owing to the number of speculators who, with or without encouragement from the man himself, played the market on Cutten's coat-tails to the tune of about one million dollars. Then all across North America were stories that Cutten and some of the other manipulators had switched from playing bull to playing bear, clearing millions and leaving everyone else to get burned. Suspicion grew that in making the gift Cutten had been trying to buy a sanctuary for use when the debacle came, or that the donation was a sort of post-dated apology to the citizens of Guelph.

Whatever the case, the hotel was a grand scheme and a wonderful magnet for favourable publicity, as when Premier Ferguson would inspect the site and comment generously. But it was to be partly a facility for the students of the agricultural college, now the University of Guelph. Since students would be benefiting, Cutten asked for the use of inmates at the Guelph provincial reformatory in order to keep costs down. The government apparently bowed to his parsimony at first but later backed down. So Cutten went ahead with the park but eliminated almost everything except the golf course, to which he retained title. Such was the initial publicity during the boom spring of 1929, however, that most Guelph residents simply assumed the course was a city park when it was in fact no such thing. Cutten's family sold it to other private interests in the late 1930s. It is still called the Cutten Club.

When Black Thursday came the public was left searching for a saviour. Perhaps the banks would step in and shore up the market?

Perhaps Cutten, Raskob, and the others should do it? But after the irreversible Crash on Black Tuesday the public became a mob and the purpose of the search to find a villain. Once again Cutten's name was on many people's lips. Cutten phoned the office of the Guelph *Daily Mercury* and denied that he was in any way responsible. He himself, he insisted, had been caught in the collapse and his own holdings had suffered significantly. But to people already well along in the search for scapegoats this answer didn't wash.

The *Toronto Daily Star* called Cutten "the Samson who pulled down the pillars of the exchange" in New York. The paper quoted unnamed Wall Street sages as saying Cutten, since September 1, had been part of the greatest bear pool ever known. His partner, the *Star* went on, was Jesse L. Livermore of Boston, who would soon issue his own denial. "What little business I have done in the stock market," he said, "has always been as an individual and will continue to be done on such a basis." On the surface the theory would seem preposterous, as Cutten and Livermore, another grain baron, were old antagonists to say the least. At the time, however, the situation was far from clear, and Cutten exerted a certain fascination, especially in Canada.

On October 25 it was reported that Cutten was dumping wheat on the Winnipeg grain market. Rumours spread that he unloaded 6 million bushels because he needed cash to cover his New York stock losses. The *Star*, however, claimed to see through a clever ruse. "Cutten was simply 'beating the public to it', in the racy description of the men behind the scenes here," the paper claimed. The big grain speculators, it seems, were all long in wheat, and also over-extended in their New York stock dealings. Cutten, according to this theory, saw their inevitable foundering. He practically gave away his own wheat to scotch any chance they would have to prop up the bull market in stocks. So, the theory ran, the NYSE came crashing down and Cutten cleaned up.

Other observers, notably the New York *Evening Journal*, refused to believe that old enemies like Cutten and Livermore could work together. The *Journal*, in common with most observers, was far more interested in whether or not Cutten had "covered" when the market broke, whether he was in fact its shrewd manipulator or another hapless victim, only with more at stake. And this was in turn all part of a general anarchy of scuttlebutt in which no one seemed able to explain why the fall had come or what would happen next. Cutten himself, the *Star* claimed, was operating from the Hotel Traymore in Atlantic City, periodically racing to New York, where a branch office of a Chicago underwriting firm kept a private room for his exclusive use.

What seems clear in retrospect is that Cutten was in no position to avoid making enemies. The Crash was the signal that the image of the businessman was slated for a drastic change. Soon bus drivers would no longer tug their forelocks and tell of having once seen some tycoon plain; they would be going to Frank Capra movies instead. Cutten's reputation was especially vulnerable because he had been looked upon by a whole section of Canadian society as one of their own. Not only had he let them down but now, Margaret Trudeau-like, he was the source of some embarrassment internationally.

A few days before the Crash, Cutten had let it be mentioned in brokers' newsletters that he was a buyer and investor in the stocks of Yellow Cab, Simmons Bed, and other companies with which his connection was, to say the least, common knowledge. On October 26 he was taken to task for this in an editorial in the Toronto *Globe*.

> Hundreds of Canadians took trading positions in that stock because of Mr. Cutten's statement, and scores are reported to have been wiped out…. Most of these have believed in the sincerity of Mr. Cutten and, therefore, are not blaming him. The *Globe* still believes that Mr. Cutten was sincere in presenting the merits of the stock. But a great deal of feeling is being excited by stories that Mr. Cutten, instead of suffering along with all the others, had been a bear all along and has been sell-

ing the stocks which he had been indirectly or directly induc-
ing others to buy.

But still no one knew for sure how large a role Cutten had played.
Cutten himself certainly had no intention of saying, given his habit
of acting mysteriously even when there was little need to do so.
("Compared to him," the *New York Times* once commented, "the
sphinx was a blatherskite.") What remains the most thorough exam-
ination came in 1930, in a book, *Mystery Men of Wall Street*, by Earl
Sparling, a New York newspaperman.

It was Sparling's contention that Cutten survived the Crash with
a fortune of as much as $80 million "without unloading his basic hold-
ings during the decline and fall of the market". His method, Sparling
claimed, was first to liquidate his previous holdings and begin borrowing. That done, he would invest millions in Radio, Monkey Ward, and
the few other favourite stocks, some of which rose to 300 or 400
points. "The remainder of his capital he used strategically over the
three-year period, buying and selling additional blocks of various
stocks, according to constantly changing conditions. Usually he sold
on a 10 or 15 point movement, whether up or down, at profit or loss.
If he won he marked the gain off the cost of his basic holdings, which
he kept always intact. If he lost he added the loss to the original cost
of these holdings." By this method he apparently repaid all his loans
and marked working profits off the cost of his original holdings. In
time he had 100,000 or even 200,000 shares each of Radio and
Monkey Ward, free and clear, without having actually put a cent toward their outright purchase. "He had changed, in other words, from
a speculator to an investor.... When the Crash came he had only to sit
tight. He had cleared his decks. He had amassed an additional fortune,
several times larger than the first one, consisting of some hundreds of
thousands of shares which had cost him nothing."

But he had remained at any event a wheeler and dealer, at first
alluring and later reviled. Sparling's book quickly sold through a
number of printings. In the rare-books room at Princeton University

is a copy once owned by Scott Fitzgerald, with underlinings and marginalia pertaining to Cutten, as though Fitzgerald planned to make him part of some fictional composite.

After the Crash, Cutten became bitter. In April 1929 he had been interviewed by the most flowery newspaper writer in Canada, the *Star*'s R. E. Knowles, a reformed clergyman who had turned to journalism after suffering a nervous breakdown. Knowles asked what advice he would give the young men of the Dominion and Cutten replied, "Work hard and do the square thing." But by 1930 his tone was different. "There has been far too much bunk in Canadian papers about my hotel plans, my stock deals, and myself," he told Knowles in January. "I am not friendly with Canadian papers. They are far too impertinent." The hardest questions, however, were being asked not in Canada but in the States.

First came revelations about Albert H. Wiggin, the head of the Chase National Bank in New York. It seems he had been receiving large retainers and director's fees from concerns eager to borrow money from the Chase. Also, he had been speculating in the market, particularly in Chase stock, with money from the bank's own vaults. Such dealings had been carried out through any of a half-dozen personal holding companies, some of them incorporated in Canada for dark reasons. One of these holding companies had engaged with Harry F. Sinclair and Arthur Cutten in boosting the stock of Sinclair and Cutten's own Consolidated Oil.

Later, the Senate Committee on Banking and Currency began a formal search for someone to take the fall for what had happened to the market. Each of the big manipulators was called in turn: Sinclair, Percy Rockefeller, Bernard E. (Sell 'em Ben) Smith. Cutten, when called, appeared to have difficulty hearing the senators' questions. A poor memory for details added to his lack of presence before the committee. At length the investigators settled for coming down hard on Richard Whitney, head of the New York Stock Exchange during the late unpleasantness. His fall came later, in an unrelated bit of nasty business, when he was tried on charges of grand larceny. At about this time, too, Sinclair finally went to jail for refusing to answer questions about his part in the 1923 Teapot Dome scandal.

As for Cutten, after 1929 he became even more of an enigma, if that's possible. He was being damned by farmers across North America for his tinkering with the price of their grain. But when the price seemed to perk up a bit in April 1933 (it was a false spring), there were some who said Cutten was behind this trend as well and should be thanked. Certainly Cutten, in his rare public remarks, tried to befriend those who derided him. A third of all the wheat, oats, and corn in the United States, he charged at one point, went "into the pockets of those who grow fat at the farmers' expense". One assumes this was Cutten the weekend farmer speaking, not King Cutten, the little giant of the pits.

He was still a figure to be watched closely. Before the Crash it had been his custom to feed two boxes of corn each day to the pigeons that gathered on the window ledge of his LaSalle Street office, but afterwards he limited himself to one box per day. Then, on April 21, 1933, he was spotted with two boxes once again, just as in the old days, and observers interpreted this as a prediction that the end of all such austerity, large and small, was at hand. Cutten himself was optimistic enough, saying more than once that soon the "economic fog will lift."

His legal troubles began in 1934. At first their scale was small. In February, a writer named John R. Mauff brought suit against him for $50,000. Mauff claimed he had worked for Cutten ghosting articles and letters to high government officials but had not been paid; Mauff won and was awarded $10,000. But then in April the federal government charged Cutten with failing to report $50 million in grain futures holdings in 1930 and 1931. It came to light that Cutten had actually made a killing by selling short while trying to have himself remembered as the farmers' bullish friend. He was ordered barred from the pits for two years, but he took the ban all the way to the Supreme Court, which ruled in his favour in May 1936.

Meanwhile he had been charged with failure to pay his full income tax in various years going back to 1929.

Cutten died in Chicago that June, aged 66. The federal government pursued the unsettled account with his estate, only to learn Cutten's total wealth amounted to a paltry $350,000, at least as far as the probate court was concerned. Eventually the U.S. authorities were able to recover more than $1 million of what was owed them, but nothing more. Shortly before his death, it was said, Cutten sold himself short, as it were; in a manoeuvre that must have hurt him in the purse but only in the short run, he was said to have transferred his assets, a reported $90 million, to Canada. He made, so to speak, a killing on his own death. Or so the story goes. Others contend he went broke like everyone else. The preference for one ending over the other is largely a question of temperament.

7

The Age of Prosperity

Floyd Chalmers likes to tell a story about an acquaintance he calls Charlie, a customer's man in one of the important Montreal brokerage houses during the bull years. Charlie spent his days executing orders on behalf of clients, who by 1929 were amassing staggering paper profits almost without effort. He saw no reason, in that largely unregulated age, why he should not do the same himself. The brokers in those days did not employ top analysts as they do today, and during the great boom especially the popularity of particular stocks was often determined by mass supposition. The run on a stock had to begin somewhere, usually with an uncharacteristic purchase, a widely circulated rumour, a gossip campaign. Charlie was in a position to have the inside track, and in what seemed like very little time he was said to be worth a million or two on paper.

One night in September that year, Charlie attended a private party. The party was quite legally "wet" as Canada was not then undergoing Prohibition as the United States was. In fact, the sale of Canadian alcohol to Americans was one of the major growth industries if also one of the least documented. About $40 million worth was being smuggled into the States annually, by one conservative (very conservative) estimate; another account suggests $2 million *per week* was changing hands at the Windsor-Detroit border just in bribes to the authorities. In any event, the festivities got out of hand, and at one point some short-skirted young women staged a contest to see who could do the highest cancan kicks. One of them accidentally kicked the customer's man in the back of the neck and he slipped into a coma from which he didn't recover until 1931. By then his millionaire status had vanished. "The last time I saw him was in Jamaica in 1933," recalls Chalmers. "He was sort of a beachcomber, greeting ocean liners and shilling for one of the hotels."

At least Charlie had an excuse. Most of the others who got wiped out were present and accounted for when the debacle began and, if they perceived the danger coming, failed to act quickly enough, if at all. Many, of course, were happy amateurs playing a game which even professionals found treacherous. There was a report in the press, for example, of a nincompoop who acquired a unique portfolio. He bought, in order, one share of each of the stocks listed alphabetically in the day's tabulation; by the time of the so-called Babson Break he had got as far as the H's and showed a profit. But then it's as easy to condemn such foolhardy speculation as it is difficult to put oneself back in the psychological state that encouraged it. It's hard to keep in mind how basic and widespread was the belief in almost unlimited economic growth. When even economists couldn't agree on the immediate future, what were mere civilians to believe? How could people be faulted for looking up to those in charge of the country's purse-strings and being reassured? Canada seemed boundless in its economic zeal.

By 1929, for example, there were three-hundred-odd people around the world carrying one million dollars or more in life insurance and several of these were Montreal and Toronto businessmen. The most heavily insured was said to be Percy Cowans, of the Montreal brokerage house of MacDougall and Cowans, whose policies totalled $1.4 million; he was later involved in a stock scandal. Colonel F. H. Deacon, a Toronto broker, was second with $1.2 million. H. C. Hatch, the president of Hiram Walker–Gooderham and Worts, the Toronto distillery, and P.C. Larkin, the Salada Tea president who orchestrated Mackenzie King's trust fund, each had policies totalling $1 million. H. C. Fox, the head of one of the country's biggest packing-houses, and Eli Dunkelman, the immigrant whose son made the family's fortune with Tip Top Tailors, didn't appear on the list, each having only $500,000 in coverage.

But the mood was not a question of this and more orthodox indicators (such as bank clearances or productivity indexes) which seem so clear in retrospect. It was a case, rather, of all the other common evidence by which people outside the money world intuitively and subconsciously judge their quality of life. Consumer goods in hand were more impressive than any graph, as in the case of automobiles. In 1929 there were more than a million passenger cars in Canada, up from fewer than five thousand only 20 years earlier; American production for the year wasn't surpassed until 1953. And the flivvers came in an almost infinite variety. The one small black car of Henry Ford seemed a long way in the past, and the present trend of compaction, by which our energy-pressed society is slowly returning to Ford's ideal, was unforeseen by even the dreamiest prophets, like the ones who that year created a new comic-strip character named Buck Rogers.

Building was another sign. A person could not help being impressed and if necessary reassured by the unprecedented construction boom, whose main impact was to be found, not in statistics on housing starts, but in the everyday cityscapes. In Ottawa, the Canadian National was enlarging by almost half the 17-year-old, 360-room Château Laurier. In Winnipeg, James Richardson was making public a scheme to erect a $3 million skyscraper at Portage and Main. Richardson, one of the Richardson Richardsons, was among the few native westerners important in the brokerage business, and a general tycoon. He founded what eventually became Air

Canada and once came within 100,000 or so shares of controlling International Nickel, which *Time* termed the "bluest of Canada's blue chips".

In Montreal, the Royal Bank put up its new headquarters on St. James Street. St. Andrew's Church, on Beaver Hall Hill, built in 1851, was pulled down so that Bell Canada, a company rightly judged to have enormous growth potential, could realize its astoundingly tall home office (20 storeys). It boasted a cinema as well as koko panelling in the boardroom and an elegant fireplace with a small marble relief of the city's true economic founder, the beaver.

But then Montreal had always *looked* wealthy. The changes were more striking in Toronto, which only a generation earlier gave the appearance of a prosperous but relatively obscure imperial outpost, its many church steeples the most visible landmarks from a distance. Now everything was booming—not *just* the churches but *even* the churches. St. Alban the Martyr was begun in a then stately residential area called the Annex, where the Eatons still kept a house. But the church had scarcely got beyond the nave stage when the Crash halted construction. On a larger scale, the same fate befell Eaton's new College Street store. Yet another near-failure was the Park Plaza Hotel, which wasn't completed until 1937. New landmarks completed under the wire were the Bank of Commerce tower and the Royal York Hotel.

This wholesale rebuilding of cities was not a localized or even a particularly Canadian phenomenon, however. As Galbraith has pointed out, most of the prominent architectural landmarks in the medium-sized cities of America date from this period. In New York, several groups were making competing plans for the world's tallest building. The eventual winning entry, the Empire State Building, was finally completed in 1931. Rockefeller Center and the Chrysler Building are also graduates of 1929. But Toronto felt itself second to none in its ambitions. Plans were tabled to completely restructure the face of King Street and University Avenue. A great hub dedicated to the memory of those who had fallen in the Great

War was to dominate the financial district, and rows of new sky-scrapers were to stand at attention.

But the district, and in fact the city as a whole, quickly went into the construction doldrums when the market swooned and stag-gered; and the scheme was abandoned. The only skyscraper spurred by the plan to actually get built was the Gothic home of the *Daily Star*, which made a famous address of 80 King Street West; the build-ing was hailed as a marvel, especially in the pages of the *Star*. And then, the end. Completion in 1949 of the Bank of Nova Scotia's art deco headquarters at King and Bay (on the site of the 1852 home of William Cawthra, one of the earliest bankers) marked the first major office building since the beginning of the Depression.

While the spirit lasted, however, the transformations were the pride of the young and a scourge to the memory of the old. Vancouver toyed with a proposal for a massive new downtown devel-opment, like Toronto's, but this was another victim. Yet there was one building put up during Vancouver's own boom that seems to symbol-ize the spirit of informed confidence. The 50-member Vancouver Stock Exchange, one of the most roguish in the country because of its closely held power and its dependence on mining, had been built only in 1907; until that time shares were traded in saloons. In the in-tervening years the exchange had occupied eight different structures, none of them adequate to the task. Then came the boom.

The city was still obviously under-industrialized, still too de-pendent on eastern and foreign capital. But this didn't seem to matter; it has been said (and not believed) that the city had 83 mil-lionaires, none of them public benefactors. Handsome buildings were going up all around, as in the case of the Royal Bank's Granville and Hastings branch. Across Howe Street from the fin-ished Hall Building, S. W. Miller, the president of the exchange, conceived the idea of a new home for the VSE. The result was a 10-storey affair of orange brick and terra cotta with a basement-to-second-floor pit and its main entrance on Pender. This was the street on which most of the brokers (the indigenous ones and branch offices of eastern biggies such as Ames, Wood Gundy, and Nesbitt Thomson) had their offices, making the term "Howe Street broker" a misnomer.

Miller's plan was to lease back space to the exchange and engage all the financial community as tenants. The building opened with great fanfare but its hopes were killed by the pandemonium of October. Before long the building was sold, and for years afterward there were squabbles about its declining tax assessment. That was not the last irony, however. At one stage in its later life the building housed the offices of the unemployment insurance commission.

Obviously a man such as Miller should have been in an excellent position to know that the bull market and the boom were coming to an end. But it's unfair to single him out for lacking the perspicacity to act. He wasn't the only one who knew better but failed to read the signs. Nor was he the only person involved in some scheme predicated on continued good health for the securities fraternity. There are indications that in 1929 the financial insiders were looking to the general businessmen for guidance rather than the other way around. Or it's at least obvious that those involved in Montreal, Toronto, and New York brokerages were, like nearly everyone else, more caught up in the spirit of the times than rational thinking entitled them to be.

As the autumn of 1929 progressed, broker and customer alike were living high off the hog. Millions went a long way when 10 pounds of sugar cost 54 cents and a men's suit at Eaton's only $35, when one Toronto wheeler-dealer could purchase the northeast corner of Bay and Bloor streets for a paltry five hundred thousand dollars. It was a monied, dressy time when a gentleman carried a walking stick and sometimes wore spats. These made him, the older he got, look like a depiction of "Capital" in some left-wing editorial cartoon. For women, skirts were still short but the cloche was being displaced by another type of hat, the cabbage leaf, which despite its name looked more like a sailor's sou'wester. Such clothes reflected a confidence, a swagger, not entirely lost on the financial community.

In New York, for instance, the nine daily newspapers all had ship's reporters. These were fellows who went out on the pilot boats to board incoming ocean liners before they docked and get interviews with returning celebrities and visiting foreign notables. By this time, however, even the *Wall Street Journal* had joined this practice. It sought interviews with travelling financiers and businessmen, who had no excuse for being uninformed after so long a journey: transatlantic liners had begun installing stock tickers and at least one featured a broker's branch office. But then the *Journal* was no doubt apprehensive about new competition, as financial journalism suddenly became more popular than ever before. With timing that was remarkably bad (or remarkably good) both *Fortune* and *Business Week* chose 1929 as their year of birth.

This was all part of the general atmosphere no less prevalent in Canada than in the United States. The fascination of wealth spans all ages and cultures, but its appeal now was almost without precedent. Partly this was because new means existed for exciting people's envy. The movies, for instance, were then at their height in terms of box office. Intrigued by the innovative talkies, an amazing 110 million Americans went to the cinema every week. The figure was down to 60 or 75 million during the depth of the Depression, when escapism, supposedly, was most avidly sought. And with the movies came the movie stars, whose quick rise to riches may have instilled the bug in people previously thought immune. Certainly money talk was everywhere, as newspapers became attentive to the movements of the well-to-do. Probate court was a dignified beat as stories about big inheritances grew common.

Such were the dreams of the man and woman in the street, and for the financial community, too, there were now entirely new types of wealth. The 19th century, after all, was only one generation gone to the young Turks of 1929. The first half of it had been dominated by the fur trade, the second half by railways. Now there were other areas, unknown to their fathers, for sober and right-thinking men in their prime. The utilities field, for example, was one that had already proved its enormous potential in Montreal and Toronto.

In the former city there were already people who, if they chose, could live off the interest on the interest from power fortunes. In 1901, for instance, Senator Louis J. Forget had gone into partnership with Herbert (later Sir Herbert) Holt to bring the existing electric and gas companies together under the umbrella of Montreal Light, Heat and Power. Forget was one of the relative handful of French-Canadian business titans (another, in later years, would be his nephew, Sir Rodolphe Forget), and his association with Holt one of the rare instances of the two founding races making a killing together. Their capitalization was $17 million, a figure that seemed stupendous at the time.

Then there was Izaak Walton Killam. He assembled power companies for such faraway romantic places as Calgary and Argentina and in doing so became one of the richest individuals in Canada. Later he bought Royal Securities from Lord Beaverbrook, who didn't need it any longer. Still another example, though not on quite the same scale, was R. O. Sweezey. He found himself at the centre of a scandal in the 1930s when his company, Beauharnois Power, was accused of having made payoffs to certain politicians.

Toronto, too, had its utilities giants, the most notable being Sir Henry Pellatt. It was Sir Henry's fate that he bore a strong resemblance to an enervated walrus. But he was so active in various branches of business that no one could doubt his being a mogul of the first order. At various times, for instance, he was heavily into mining, shipping, and meat-packing; he was also one of the directors of the infamous Home Bank when it collapsed in 1923. But the basis of all this was electricity. Sir Henry was one of those who had the idea that a bloody fortune could be made controlling the lines on which hydro-electric power was carried a hundred miles from Niagara Falls to Toronto. His privately owned Electrical

Development Company was eventually taken over by Ontario Hydro, a Crown corporation.

In 1911, after making his fortune, Pellatt began construction of a Toronto home he called Casa Loma. It was a mansion of 98 rooms, 30 bathrooms (including some with gold fixtures), 25 fireplaces, 3 bowling alleys, a shooting gallery... the list is only a partial one. To design it he retained E. J. Lennox, whose public buildings, including the old City Hall, have now overshadowed his role as builder to the private elite; he was, for instance, the family architect of the Masseys in all but actual title. Pellatt had very definite ideas of what he wanted, having studied the castles of Europe. The result has been called a mixture of 17th-century Scottish baronial and 20th Century Fox. The structure was completed in 1914, after which Lennox retired from architecture, as though from embarrassment. But Casa Loma's life as a private residence was brief. By 1924 Pellatt was short of money and moved out. Two unsuccessful attempts were made to operate it as a hotel but by the time of the Crash its fate was sealed.

If by that time the financial world seemed to have turned completely upside down, this doesn't detract from the usefulness of Pellatt and the others as symbols. There was, to be sure, a general rush of at times disbelieving confidence so far as the market was concerned. In Canada, the sensation reached its height with regard to a whole category of stocks—or rather, a whole group of industries which men such as Pellatt represented, in their capacity as the country's first indigenous castle-builders. In pulp and paper the biggies were Abitibi, Price Brothers, Spanish River, Wayagamack, and Howard Smith. In the automobile field there was Russell Motor Car and also Carriage Factories Limited. And in power, in addition to the ones just named, there was Shawinigan Water and Power and of course Brazilian Traction, Light and Power. One or two other categories were equally strong. But there was nothing like the variety of today, with large retailing chains, oil giants, and high technology companies. Physically, too, the markets were much different.

For the Montreal Stock Exchange, as for so much else in Canadian society at the time, the Great War had been a kind of point of no return. At one time the exchange was a clubby place. Membership was limited by bylaw to only 40 people, who were known, not often affectionately, as the Forty Thieves. It later began spreading its power around, though there was no mistaking it for an open shop. The incredible boom in the years before the war had made everyone rich. In 1901, a seat cost an average of $12,850; by 1908 the figure had more than doubled, to $27,500. This may seem picayune by the standards of early and mid 1929, when seats went for about $225,000. But the jump seemed more enormous then, coming as it did so quickly.

During the war the exchange was closed down, like Toronto's. It reopened to find a recession and then finally the first signs of the coming boom years. Yet the war years were the watershed. In 1919, for instance, over 900,000 shares were traded one day, while pre-Crash trading for 1929 averaged 250,000. Until the Crash with its Black Thursday and Black Tuesday, the public simply had no short-hand for separating the good times from the bad. It was the war that loomed large in the imagination, as a dark time that had interrupt-ed the natural, *orderly* economic flow. People with their wits about them were beginning to realize something else as well: that only since the war had Toronto started to become a serious rival in mat-ters of finance.

The MSE building in rue St-François-Xavier (as it was almost never called in those days) was only 26 years old at the time of the great stock calamity. It still had a lot of life left in it, and in fact wasn't abandoned for newer premises until 1965. Yet it seemed an ancient place even then, the formality and staidness of its occupants giving it a kind of instant tradition. This ersatz timelessness was much envied by the Toronto Stock Exchange, whose members did their best to be bluenoses but were often made to feel upstarts by comparison. Sir Herbert Holt could throw inquiring newspaper-men down the stairs, as he was reputed to do, and still come out shining, while they themselves were haunted by the presence of the notorious Standard mining exchange a few blocks away.

Make no mistake about it, Toronto was a wide-open town financially despite the presence of brokers whose seats had been handed down through the family from the time when membership had cost only five dollars. There was financial razzmatazz in the air in those days, and one of the best ways to recapture the feeling is through the press. The *Daily Star* and the *Evening Telegram* covered business the way they covered everything: sensationally. The *Globe* was the tamest of the lot. But the paper most concerned with money matters was the *Globe*'s rival, the *Mail and Empire*, a peculiar mixture of financial news and reports of bizarre crimes. In Montreal, by comparison, the *Star* was perhaps a bit wilder than the *Gazette*, though this was a fine distinction. Neither covered the stock markets the way Toronto thought they ought to be covered. Montreal just didn't have all of Toronto's mining activity to lure charlatans, excite the public's greed, and generally stir matters up. Neither did it have all the superstructure typified by two very dissimilar tabloid-sized papers called *Hush* and the *Northern Miner*.

Hush, which first appeared in 1928, was a scandal sheet with a special fondness for Bay Street stories which would have been unprintable anywhere else, though its sexual references are what endeared it to two or three generations of Canadian and foreign readers. The *Northern Miner* was very different. This curious weekly had been another product of the Cobalt silver rush. It had been founded in 1915 by two northern newspapermen on, according to legend, an initial capitalization of $10. Soon they were bought out by the three Pearce brothers under the leadership of Norman Pearce, later known as "the Colonel". (The 1920s were littered with colonels, as the generation that first over-achieved in the Great War was just then settling down to business, but Pearce's eventual title dated from the Second World War.) In 1928, the brothers saw the pattern unfolding and moved the paper to Toronto. It was more important for them to be close to the principal raw material—small investors—than to the mines themselves. They were frequently to be seen in the Standard building on Richmond Street and at the loftier TSE on Bay, which despite its inferiority complex had come to have a certain tradition of its own.

The Greek-style building with its huge columns stood at 84-86 Bay Street on a site purchased from Sir Henry Pellatt for $153,000. It had opened in 1913 and members were comfortably settled in time for the exchange to be closed by government order the following year. But the suspension lasted only three months, and in no time the exchange was secreting a folklore which for years would be passed on by word of mouth, at least within a radius of a few blocks.

Everyone loved recalling the story of a pixyish broker who purchased twenty thousand shares of Continental Kirkland at one-eighth of a cent to mail out with his Christmas cards. Soon after he finished posting the last batch the price rose to 80 cents per share—a 640-fold appreciation. And for years the exchange had a permanent resident: a nameless cat who became a sort of good-luck charm. It was widely believed that mining stocks shot up every time she gave birth to a litter, which she (and they) did frequently. But this was later. The cat was still alive, for instance, in 1937 when the exchange moved into its present building, the first totally air-conditioned commercial structure in Canada. Although on almost the same site as the old building, the current one is No. 237 Bay, owing to an official renumbering of the street. However, old 84-86 was still new, and felt new, when the troubles began in 1929. But it aged very quickly in October of that year.

The fatal month began happily enough, though the markets were still jittery after the dramatic events of September. In Toronto, prices were generally depressed. In Montreal, the *Gazette* navel-gazed its list of 20 representative issues and concluded that, on the basis of September, the index "would suggest a period of steadily declining prices." But such predictions were common at moments like these. There was still no mass acceptance of the fact that disaster lay three weeks away. Quite the contrary.

A general sense of satisfaction underlay the momentary nervousness. In Montreal, construction was setting records, even though in the United States, according to a Canadian Press report on the subject, "preoccupation with stock market speculation was blamed for the slump" in building which that country was beginning to experience. It was announced that Canadian companies would be paying out an unprecedented amount of dividends during the month (more than $32 million, with the CPR heading the list at $9.6 million). So the future was still bright. Cries to the contrary seemed faraway or unimportant or quibbling, as when a committee investigating British banking professed alarm at North American speculation and when Grand Duke Alexandr Michaelovich, the deposed czar's brother-in-law, told a Montreal suffrage group that he saw "an over-emphasis on materialism".

Later there were two tremors in the market which seem far less significant in retrospect than at the time. Even shortly afterward, in fact, it was accepted that, as the *Gazette* put it, "the stocks on Canadian markets gave a good account of themselves." The reasoning ran that prices were a bit inflated anyway, and these small adjustments were just that—adjustments. There was also the popular theory that should call money on Wall Street drop to 5 per cent, a lot of Canadian funds would be repatriated. This would boost the Canadian dollar (then about 99 cents U.S.), which had not benefited as usual from foreign purchases of wheat, as most of the crop was still in storage. But then again, as the *Daily Star* in Toronto observed, such remarks were being made cautiously. "The experts have been wrong so often lately that they are more reticent about expressing an opinion."

For experts read economists and other theoretical soothsayers. The actual leaders of the financial community were pushing forward as usual. On October 12, a thousand American investment bankers left Grand Central Station in two special trains bound for their annual convention in Quebec City. They were in a confident mood. On the 15th, 30 of the brightest young men in the Toronto financial world assembled to found the exclusive Ticker Club, which still exists. They too viewed the future positively. Ten days followed and the late Colonel W. H. Jolliffe, then another young man starting out, conducted his first full day of business as a member of the Toronto Stock Exchange, where seats were now selling for $220,000, or almost as much as in Montreal. But in that last 10-day period the world had collapsed. Jolliffe was too late. Twenty-four hours earlier the system had caved in.

8

The Crash

As the third week of October got under way there was unspoken agreement that conditions were getting better, scattered bad news notwithstanding. In Britain, the financial empire of Clarence Hatry had fallen apart. This put a momentary kibosh on North American confidence as foreign speculators sold out in order to cover themselves. Then, in Boston, the state public-utilities board had refused to sanction a stock split by the Edison Company. This, too, did passing harm to Wall Street. It probably also wiped out the public-relations gains being made by the company; the corporation had been celebrating the 50th anniversary of the invention of the incandescent bulb by Thomas Edison, who also, incidentally, perfected the stock printer. Generally, though, the mood was roseate until Wednesday the 23rd, the date of the biggest break so far—the one that put a terrible scare in even the most boosterish market-watchers.

All the eastern bourses opened at 10 a.m. It wasn't long afterward that the New York Stock Exchange ticker began to lag behind amid heavy trading, thus adding frustration to the situation in Canada. The main Toronto and Montreal exchanges were not connected to one another by ticker until 1931 but made do with discontinuous telephone reports and the brokers' own wires. This left them even more sensitive to developments in Wall Street than they would have been otherwise, and sometimes inconsistent as well. In the morning, for example, Montreal briefly held firm and later appeared to be moving downward only at the same velocity as in the past few days. But brokers in Toronto, it appears, had more success in maintaining communication with the big board in New York and therefore got worse news more quickly.

At noon that day the Montreal Lions Club met at the Mount Royal Hotel to hear William W. Goforth, research director at Cockfield, Brown and Company, the advertising agency, deliver an address entitled "The Economic Outlook of Canada". He considered the future would be bright despite the possibility of a temporary slowdown in 1930, which in any event would be nothing compared to the stock market dip of May 1920. Some time around 2:30, when it became apparent to the financial community that New York was really bracing itself for a full panic, a corresponding shock was felt here. Three of the most popular Canadian stocks—International Nickel, Brazilian Traction, and Hiram Walker—were interlisted on the New York exchange. Local brokers therefore knew at once, by private wire, when the trio broke in New York. There was an immediate reaction in Toronto, where these issues were dumped in lots of from 200 to nearly 1,000 shares. They dropped a combined 8¼ points.

Of other high-volume stocks, only Noranda rose that day on the TSE and this gain was attributed to the announcement that morning of a new mining venture. Otherwise, the big stocks—except the oils—were down, a great number hitting record lows for the year. In Montreal, the outcome was almost identical save for the fact the paper and power companies generally stood their ground. Only a few bears were reported to have done well but they must have been few indeed.

The volume of trading was staggering, and this alone was enough to catapult the whole situation from the financial sections of the newspapers to the front pages. Of course, the effect of the break on local markets was the angle journalists preferred. The Calgary *Herald* ran an editorial lamenting not just the devaluation of stocks but the concurrent fall in wheat prices. In Winnipeg, too, it was naturally this second concern that seemed most pressing. The best insight belonged to the *Mail and Empire*. "The inability of the New York ticker to keep pace with the falling market," it reported, "may have saved some of the locals from a more serious punishment." It reasoned that since the New York quotations were as much as an hour behind the reality, and the Toronto board somewhat behind that, there was little time *left* for a panic in Toronto. But no doubt this would only prejudice opening prices tomorrow.

Still to be heard from was the *Financial Post*, which appeared to be testing the tensile strength of its metaphor: "The man who eventually is apt to find himself in a satisfactory position is the one who has trimmed his sails to the prevailing winds and guided his barque into the less turbulent waters that lie in close proximity to the shore. This is no time for anyone to steer one's course into the open." This sage advice, however, didn't appear on the news-stands until the following day, October 24. Once again, the *Post* was at a disadvantage in trying to cover daily events on a weekly basis. For the 24th was Black Thursday, when advice, regardless how good, ceased being worth much.

All through the night brokers had been calling their customers, telling them to put up more margin immediately or be sold out. Many had no choice but to forfeit. But despite this situation and the general tension carried over from Wednesday, the markets opened pretty steadily, though the volume of trading was enormous right from the start. In New York, several blue chips sold in blocs as big as twenty thousand shares. The selling orders kept pouring in so quickly that there was no chance of the tape's staying up to date even for a short time. Before the market was open a full hour it was obvious that this was, in the patois of the gangster movie, curtains.

Later commentators would attempt to allot parts of the day to various psychological types: the margin traders who were first to sell, followed by the panic sellers, with the short sellers somewhere in between perhaps. If it is difficult to pinpoint such matters from a distance, it was next to impossible at the time, so great was the mêlée.

In Montreal, on both the senior exchange and the Curb, the panic was almost unrestrained. The greatest chaos was caused by brokers emptying their customers' portfolios. Total sales would reach almost 400,000 shares on the MSE, an absolutely unprecedented figure; by noon almost every stock on the board had lost anywhere up to 25 points. In Toronto, it was almost impossible to get a bid. Losses went up to 10, 15, and even 20 points in a few cases. Among the hardest hit were Loblaws, Steel Company of Canada, Consolidated Bakeries, and Canada Gypsum—all the tried-and-true safe stocks. Even Brazilian and that old standby, International Nickel, dropped markedly in a few minutes; Massey-Harris sank to within a point of matching the lowest price in its history, and some others were not even that lucky. At noon, the Toronto Stock Exchange's own ticker was running behind, a rare occurrence.

At almost exactly that same moment two events were unfolding in New York. Inside the NYSE at Wall and Broad streets, the exchange's acting president, Richard Whitney, made the decision to clear the visitors' gallery. Only a few months earlier the exchange had announced proudly that visitors were up 50 per cent over summer 1928. But already this morning seven hundred people had jammed inside the 7-foot-wide deck that looked across to the wall-sized mechanical ticker, to the Big Board at the far right and the general chaos 20 feet below. "Some onlookers wept and others screamed—," Robert Sobel has written, "while the brokers themselves were in tears and hoarse with shouting."

There are conflicting stories about whether Whitney was only concerned about the possibility of riot or whether he actually feared the balcony of the 26-year-old building might collapse. Before the tourists and visitors could be shooed out, they had already witnessed the destruction of about $9 billion in paper wealth. Once outside they mingled with the even bigger throng in the street. The police were now maintaining order within the crowd, which seemed to have gathered for no other reason than that people sensed tragedy was in the air.

While this was happening some individuals in that sea of over-coats and snap-brim hats recognized the figure of Charles E. Mitchell, the bullish president of the National City Bank, entering the office of J. P. Morgan and Company at 23 Wall Street, kitty-corner from the exchange. In a short while Mitchell was followed by representatives of the other big institutions: Albert H. Wiggin of the Chase National, Seward Prosser of Bankers Trust, and William Potter of Guaranty Trust. George F. Baker, Jr., another First National exec-utive, was already awaiting them in the office of Thomas W. Lamont, a Morgan partner. Within the span of a further few minutes this group of men, who controlled a total of more than $6 billion in as-sets, worked out an extraordinary agreement. They would ante up a total of between $20 million and $30 million to keep the market from falling apart completely and perhaps irreparably.

In the past, when old J. P. had been alive, the House of Morgan had more than once interceded in this way, but always on a much smaller scale, of course, during smaller panics. These were the city's leading financial brains; they knew at once that this time was unlike anything ever seen before. The investment trusts that were supposed to prop up depressed prices were nowhere to be found. Nor were the bargain-hunters who had always materialized during past crashes.

Desperation made the committee amazingly efficient. The bankers quickly agreed to use the pool to prop up prices where possible, particularly those of the big industrial polestars, rather than attempt fixing price levels. They separated. Lamont remained long enough to tell reporters, in one of the most famous under-statements in the history of the language, "There has been a little distress selling on the stock market."

But reporters weren't needed to convey news of the meeting to the trading floor. The jam-packed conditions made the rumour travel even more swiftly and its good effects were apparent in a very short time, with United States Steel leading the way in a small rally. Rumour alone, however, could no more save the day than it could do lasting damage. Knowledgeable marketeers waited for the tangible manifestation of the bankers' strategy. They got it about 1:30 when Whitney (a Morgan broker as well as an exchange official) assumed the unlikely role of jitney.

In stock market parlance, a jitney was a member of the exchange who bought and sold stocks on behalf of nonmember brokers in return for 50 per cent of the commission. Although the practice was the subject of periodic debate, it was widespread throughout the 1920s and not confined to marginal operators. Wood Gundy, for example, had no seat in Toronto and so jitneyed through firms that had. Now Whitney was in theory performing the same service for the banks. He began at the post where United States Steel was traded and learned that the bid had been 205; he then bid that amount for 10,000 shares, buying only 200 shares and leaving the remainder in the hands of a specialist who did nothing but buy and sell Steel all day. He proceeded to duplicate the process for each of as many as 20 other stocks until, in all, he had offered to buy $20 million or so worth of key securities. It was obvious whom Whitney was representing, and confidence was quickly stabilized. Although there was some backsliding in prices in the final hour before the closing gong sounded, the House of Morgan's daring move had worked. Steel actually closed two points higher than it had the previous day. The others were way down in price, but at least the serious rout was not the massacre it might otherwise have become.

Still, it was the worst single day in financial history to date. Less than two years earlier, Wall Street had been prophesying the time when trading might reach 5 million shares in one day; on Black Thursday the total was nearly 13 million. There had never been anything quite like this before. Restaurateurs in the financial district normally served only breakfast and lunch. Now they were placing rush orders for huge quantities of food and rounding up all available staff. It was obvious that brokerage employees would be working late over the piles of accumulated paperwork. It was 7:08 before the ticker fell silent, signalling the full extent of what remained to be done.

The swirl of unwarranted rumour was one of the most damaging forces that day. For the first time, panic was wholesale; it took in other walks of life and spread to other cities, even to other countries. There were wild stories that troops were keeping a mob in check outside the exchange building and that the pits in Buffalo and Chicago had been ordered shut. From out of nowhere came the completely untrue story that 11 brokers had just killed themselves (this is probably what started the Wall Street window-jumping image on the way to mythology). Had the rumours that day expanded to include a Martian invasion there would have been people to believe such a thing had really happened.

This abundance of misinformation at the actual scene of the panic could only make matters more chaotic in Canada. With the New York ticker useless, the telegraph backed up, and open phone lines scarce, local traders did the best they could, but were naturally later than their American counterparts in separating the true from the untrue and reacting to Whitney's shoring-up techniques. There would be tales of individual heartbreak and imprudence. One broker told the *Daily Star* how customers "got in a blue funk and sacrificed good, bad and indifferent stocks with slight regard for critical analysis of the situation or the intrinsic values of their holdings." That is, they went to pieces. But one young man was reported calm, if downcast, after losing two-thirds of a six-thousand-dollar inheritance from his aunt. By late afternoon both Montreal and Toronto, apparently independent of each other for the most part, were growing steadier, though conditions were still bad when the smoke cleared. The sheer volume gave everyone the willies. The way blue chips had fallen was enough to make the ruthless weep.

On the MSE, Montreal Power, Brazilian, and International Nickel were down a total of more than $12, though these had been the first to recover; the average loss on a list of twenty stocks was $3.45. The big loser was Consolidated Smelters, which fell an incredible $35 to close at $325. The various curb markets and the Standard had all reacted in acute sympathy. In Winnipeg, wheat fell a dime a bushel in three minutes and later tumbled a further 5 cents, resisting the salvage efforts of big buyers and wiping out the small speculators. Because of the time difference, wheat had a shorter recovery period and regained only 6 cents when trading was halted for the day.

The next day, Friday the 25th, saw a change for the better on all fronts. But the change was mainly of atmosphere. The trading floors were characterized by that kind of stupefied calm one feels after great catastrophes. Selling remained dangerously voluminous but prices for the most part stubbornly refused to deteriorate any further. In New York, with a mixture of dread and curiosity, the bankers' pool was gingerly unloading some of the blocs acquired 24 hours earlier. By now, communications were more or less restored. Accurate news of the daring stop-gap operation had reached everyone concerned by the time the market opened. This had a settling effect.

Naturally there was residual fear. In the first few hours of trading in Toronto, for instance, stocks were freely dumped. But experts, echoing the sentiment of the *Wall Street Journal* that Black Thursday had been a "gamblers' panic", felt many of the vendors were out-of-town speculators acting on the rebound. There was also some distress selling due to the thousands of margin calls brokers had spent the night sending out. The blue-chip, high-volume stocks, which had taken the worst drubbing, now made the best comeback.

In Montreal, the market opened firmly, slipped a cog at the noon hour, but strengthened noticeably in the last three hours. The end result, however, was the same as in Toronto. Everyone was looking for reassurance while fearing the truth might be too harsh. "After a smash of such proportions," wrote the *Gazette*, "one is just a bit diffident in speaking of reassuring developments coming in conjunction with the day's schedule, but a survey of the situation would suggest" that reassurance was indeed called for. There was certainly no shortage of soothing statements by people in authority.

Edgar M. Smith, the chairman of the MSE, was typical, pointing out that all the brokerage houses themselves had survived intact. Smith prudently avoided the condition of the actual traders, however. Prominent bankers were kept busy fielding calls from the press. They responded with the cool detachment expected of them, though many could not resist a bit of I-told-you-so. The president of the Toronto Stock Exchange, C. E. Abbs, of A. E. Ames and Company, stated that "considering everything that happened in the New York market I think we may conservatively say that the Toronto market did not give a bad account of itself." He then made what would come to seem a curious addition to his remarks. "Fundamentally," he said, "conditions are sound in Canada...."

For some reason never satisfactorily explained, many prominent figures trying to hearten their countrymen used almost precisely these same words. Also on that day, for instance, President Herbert Hoover informed the American people, in what became a Bartlett-quality quotation, that "the fundamental business of the country, that is, production and distribution of commodities, is on a sound and prosperous basis." A. B. Mackenzie, the general manager of the Bank of Montreal, put it this way: "General conditions in the country are fundamentally sound." His opposite number at the Royal, Morris W. Wilson, said, "Fundamentally, business conditions are sound and there is no reason for pessimism.... It is well that in times like these we should not overlook the general soundness of the Canadian situation." A third chartered bank president merely inverted the sentiment and changed the focus: "There is nothing fundamentally wrong with the Canadian securities markets." In a short time, the words "fundamentally sound" would become a North American catch phrase. Gene Tunney knocked out Jack Dempsey, people would joke, but Dempsey was fundamentally sound. Flat on his back and unconscious, mind you, but fundamentally sound.

There had been some talk in New York and even in Toronto that the markets might have to remain closed on Saturday the 26th, not as a cooling-off but as a catching-up period. Clerks were working long into the night trying to reduce the accumulated paperwork. They could took forward to eating dinner at their desks Sunday evening and perhaps much of the coming week.

But trading did in fact resume on Saturday morning. Conditions proved as wobbly and inconclusive as those of Friday had been, save for a worrisome dip toward the end of the day. The pattern of assurance and doubt was repeated in print and in private conversations but now there was a subtle change in diction on the part of those who really knew the market and its ways. One had to be astute to notice the different intonation, perhaps, and to realize that some of the numbness had worn off and been replaced by something worse. On Sunday, many ministers delivered sermons on the recent events, usually of a cautionary nature. Sunday newspapers in the States printed comforting statements by a fresh batch of experts. Many of them also carried the advertisement of a large Boston investment house which began: "S-T-E-A-D-Y". Throughout the day a new fear seemed to be gaining momentum, fed partly by the unresolved decline of late Saturday. When the markets opened Monday morning these forebodings were seen to have been justified.

As soon as trading commenced the selling began. Additional margin calls had gone out by the thousands over the weekend. But in a very short time it was impossible to determine exactly what had touched off the dumping. All the elements of the previous Thursday were present. Volume in the end was only about two-thirds as heavy but the losses were even worse. Many key issues lost anywhere from 30 to almost 50 points; the *New York Times* industrials index was down 49 points. There were the crazy rumours, too. This is when the tale started that Arthur Cutten and Jesse Livermore had formed an evil alliance. There was talk that the White House was in an uproar and there were still more ghoulish suicide stories. None of this gossip was accurate. Neither, unfortunately, was the story about the bankers repeating their Thursday miracle. At 1:10 p.m. Mitchell was once again seen entering the House of Morgan. At least many people believed it was Mitchell and that this was his mission; it's been suggested that if Mitchell did in fact go there it was probably to seek a personal emergency loan.

In less than an hour such rumours made the floor more of a madhouse than it otherwise would have been. But this time no Whitney appeared to save the day, and those who had been holding back jettisoned their stocks for what they would fetch. In the last hour alone 3 million shares were sold.

At 4:30, after the exchange had closed, the bankers did in fact hold another meeting, remaining cloistered until 6:30. When they reappeared they had some not entirely pessimistic but maddeningly vague words for the press. And that was all. The banking cabal had decided there could be no repetition of their previous actions. The time had come for even them to sell what they had. That they waited as long as they did is probably all that prevented Black Tuesday from having gone down in history as Black Monday instead. Now there was little reason for anyone *not* to panic. Terror seemed the appropriate response to the situation when trading resumed the following day, October 29, 1929.

C. W. Stollery, a floor trader at the TSE, had been returning to his office late Monday afternoon when he met an acquaintance, Jack Meggeson, of Hickey, Meggeson and Company. They had exchanged pleasantries. "It was pretty bad today," Stollery had said grimly. "Yes," Meggeson had replied, "and it will be worse tomorrow." For years to come the two men would recall this brief conversation not with pride in their clairvoyance but with amazement at the depth of their understatement. When the markets opened at 10 Tuesday morning it was apparent that this was the crash. There was no up and down this time, no shoring up of prices. From the start there was little of anything but panic. This was the day that proved all the doom-sayers wrong. The doom-sayers had never been pessimistic enough.

Overnight the brokers had sent out still more margin calls and many people had made up their minds to throw in the towel. Nerves were frayed and faces transfixed with fear. Even before the first sale was recorded it was obvious that prices were plummeting. International Nickel, for instance, had fallen 9 points during the night. Once again, the ticker quickly became useless; such communications as came from New York were by way of private telegraph lines in brokers' offices. But this time being out of touch didn't seem to matter. The pandemonium was simultaneous in all the various centres as terrified investors unloaded their stocks by the job lot.

By 11:30 some 3 million shares had already been sold on the New York Stock Exchange. By noon the figure was 8 million. At that juncture the NYSE governing committee called an emergency meeting to decide whether or not the exchange should be closed. To keep from fomenting even more rumours the 40 governors assembled in a room underneath the exchange floor rather than in their ordinary conference area. They were careful to arrive in groups of no more than three. Two J. P. Morgan and Company men also attended. The room was small and didn't have enough chairs, so the committee men stood or perched on tables. They decided to keep the exchange open. They could hear the commotion coming through the ceiling. The din, in fact, was audible throughout a two-block area.

It's difficult describing the noise of the trading floor to someone who has never been to one of the major exchanges. Even on a dull day, the combined talking, calling, and shouting of several hundred people rises in a great cacophony and stays there, never varying in pitch. This day the noise was the loudest of all but did not seem unemotional and mechanical as before; it seemed to be a sound of terror like that heard in a slaughterhouse. The TSE had a cork floor which was supposed to muffle the sound, but this morning it was like a sponge that couldn't absorb any more. Customers filled the street outside, the corridors, the gallery, and the brokers' offices where numbers already irrelevant continued to be chalked up, as though only for appearances' sake. "Thank goodness I was cleaned out last Thursday," one poor devil was overheard to say with enviable calmness of tone. Almost everyone else on the floor—the traders and the exchange employees—seemed to be going crazy. Among them was Gordon Bongard, who had become a floor trader seven years earlier when he was only 23.

> By this time there was a hell of a roar and it was pretty smoky, so it was awfully hard on your voice. What you'd do was just go around the floor yelling, for instance, "Nickel going at 50!" And then soon it was "Nickel going at 49½!" and so on. It was hard to find a buyer because everybody wanted to get out fast. Anyway, it was noisy and confusing and a lot of mistakes were being made in the rush. At times there might be two or three different prices being quoted in different corners of the room. When we made a sale we were supposed to fill out a slip and get the buyer to initial it and then turn it over to an exchange employee who would look after getting it on the tape. But a lot of the slips ended up getting lost or not being filled out properly.

In Montreal one trader nearly had his clothes ripped off by the throng that rushed past him going nowhere. At all the exchanges people were reported to be weeping openly. One man fainted in a Toronto broker's office; the other customers carried him to a table in the backroom and resumed their despondent vigil in front of the board as though nothing had happened. Switchboards at the newspaper offices were jammed by anxious callers and some who actually seemed hysterical. Many felt the *Mail and Empire* would have the best information and repeatedly asked for Elgin 4401 but couldn't get through. In Winnipeg and Vancouver the scene was almost as chaotic.

Part of the problem at all these different venues was a system of communication primitive by today's standards. In 1929 efficiency still depended upon slips of paper and these went astray in the confusion. Typical was the system of the Standard, as recalled by Bill Townsend, who was 19 at the time of the Crash:

> There were trading booths, or posts as they were called, with certain stocks traded at each one. Inside each booth was a lad with a microphone. He would be handed the trading tickets and then would read the information to the boys with earphones who were marking up the big board—about ninety feet long and with a winding staircase up to it. They would mark up the bid and asked. Then the person in the booth would send the tickets on to the sorters, one of whom was me. The trading figures went up on the board but weren't listed on the post itself. So everything hinged on the floor slip.

But during the thick of it slips were being torn, mislaid, and lost. (At day's end in New York one broker found a waste-basket full of selling orders which had been misplaced and never executed.) The Standard's young men in their dark mauve tunics were in a frantic state. "Smoking was banned from time to time," Townsend recalls. "But now things were really hectic and people were bumping into one another in the thick smoke. It was pretty grim and there were a lot of long faces. Everyone wanted to sell but there were almost no bids. So, to be fair, they put all the brokers' names in a hat and drew one out whenever a bid came in." Ralph Longbottom, in later years the floor manager at the TSE, was then one of the Standard's post clerks sitting in the octagonal booths. "The traders were shouting themselves hoarse," he remembers. "Anybody who had a bid would just get bombarded as soon as he opened his mouth."

By 1:30 the volume at the New York exchange had exceeded 12 million shares. Someone (in legend, a messenger boy) jokingly offered one dollar a share for White Sewing Machine and succeeded in the absence of any other offers; only 24 hours earlier the stock had been priced at 11¼, which was itself quite a decline from its peak of

48. In Montreal, where the tumult was clearly audible for half a block, boys in red and blue blazers continued carrying order slips for the weary brokers, who would rush out in the centre of the floor and shout. A wire clerk in Solloway and Mills' office in Toronto sat as he had for hours, taking selling orders from the firm's western branches—there was a special little "dash" that translated as "sell at the market". He usually then typed the messages on a form. But today there wasn't time. He scrawled them with a pencil as quickly as he could but still could not catch up; his right hand was blistered at the end of the day. On its own wire, United Press was transmitting a report about men appearing in Wall and Broad streets with sandwich boards offering money to lend on jewellery and watches. For though buyers were scarce that day some brokers were refusing buying orders unless given cash up front. "It's more than a stock market panic," one member of the TSE said, unaware how accurate his remark was. "It's a world tragedy."

When the closing gong sounded in New York at 3 p.m., a cheer went up inside the building. But it was only a cheer of relief that at last the carnage had ended for the day. The 5 p.m. edition of the *Toronto Daily Star* bore an eight-column streamer right below the nameplate: "STOCK PRICES CRASH EARLY; SLIGHT RALLY LATER". Even this, however, was putting the best possible face on the situation. But then the papers' communications had suffered as the exchanges' had done, though the newsboys did a land-office business all the same.

Traffic became a nightmare in the financial district of Montreal, with two thousand cars jostling for parking spaces. Taxis clotted sections of the city usually deserted after five; restaurants remained open and popcorn butchers made a killing. In Toronto, limousines were seen unloading passengers on King and Bay until midnight, for this time the big traders had been mortally wounded along with the little fellows. Chauffeurs were instructed to wait while their guvs went inside to cover their margins—assuming they were able. Brokerage employees themselves worked away furiously until at least 2 a.m., trying to make order of the disorder.

Gold Diggers of 1929

At about that same hour one Montreal speculator was hailing a cab for himself and his friends. They had all been out getting drunk after the day's fiasco. Now they needed the hack to go to St. Joseph's Oratory. It was their hope that prayer would accomplish what hootch had failed to do. In Toronto, one investor arrived home with some news for his wife. He had, he said, resigned from six of the seven clubs to which they belonged, sold their second car, advertised for someone to rent the garage, and cancelled most of the family's charge accounts. That said, he fired the maid and went to bed. What else was a gentleman to do?

9

Coup de Grâce

At 11:15 a.m. on October 30, thirty or forty people came running out of a broker's office on Toronto's King Street with tears in their eyes. A crowd soon gathered, thinking the market had just fallen further. Actually, the people, most of them elderly, were the victims of a tear-gas bomb planted by some prankster. But passersby would not have been surprised if their first guess had been the correct one, since when it was all over the figures proved again how astoundingly bad the situation was. A total of 62 Canadian stocks had plunged to their lowest level of the year. International Nickel was off 10 points and Brazilian 11 points; a combined $197 million had been wiped off the market valuation of just these two unsinkable companies. The total for the *Daily Star*'s index of 16 key stocks was $1.1 billion; on Monday alone this list was devalued by $300 million, or about $1 million per minute. At a time when a million was a staggering sum this was financial destruction on an entirely new scale which brought in its aftermath a new sort of confusion.

To look at the newspapers and public records for the period immediately following the Crash is to get some sense of just how unsettled the situation must have appeared. The event itself was over now and the facts were quickly coming to light. The variable was the big one of interpretation. To the *Mail and Empire* "the punishment did not appear to be due to intrinsic conditions in Canada but to the fact that Canadian securities cannot move independently of the big boards." Surely it got no argument on that score. Nor was it any longer a simple matter of putting the blame on sinister figures trying to manipulate Wall Street. "It would be wrong to say that the bears were in control," theorized one *Toronto Daily Star* writer. "There was nobody in control...."

Despite such reports a crackpot chorus could still be heard. Many people actually believed, in those first few days after the disaster, that the Crash could be traced to events in Brussels; it seems that the previous day the Belgian market had experienced a selling wave, news of which reached North America before the opening in New York. Today this strikes us as a far-fetched dismissal of the obvious. But in such an accusatory atmosphere cool heads were necessarily at a premium. Although British and European markets had gone down this time on New York's coat-tails, the distance from the scene of the crime was perhaps sufficient to give them a certain perspective. The *Financial Times* of London was about the only organ to see the Wall Street collapse immediately for what it was, as the end of not just the fabulous bull market but the Coolidge-Hoover era of prosperity. Much more typical, alas, was the reaction of the *Financial Post*, which felt "the present stock market situation does not seem to presage a severe business depression."

Nor did the *Post* stand alone in wagging its finger at the public. "For some months the *Post* has advised its readers to keep one foot on the shore," it editorialized. "Recently those who have kept both feet on the shore have done even better than those who merely kept one foot on the shore.... One man remarked this week, 'I told you this was going to happen; I've been saying it for five years.' But the advances in security values during the past five years have been tremendously greater than the losses of the current year.... Canada will be all right." Canada would not be all right, of course, but at least the paper was correct on one point. There was indeed a lot of brilliant hindsight mixed in with the fear, the gloating, and the obstinate gossip, though all these elements tended toward one vast jumble of information.

Almost immediately after the Crash itself, there sprang up a complicated web of rumour as to who had been wiped out and who had not. Eddie Cantor, the entertainer, was ruined (he would later publish a book of favourite stock market jokes). Cyrus Eaton, the expatriate Canadian industrialist, was said to have lost $100 million. But it was presumed by the tattlers, if only later substantiated by sources close to the man himself, that old Sir Herbert Holt had, as usual, not suffered. He had not availed himself of leverage but gambled, apparently, on a relatively small scale and always with cash on hand. Not that a man who controlled as much as he did, what with the Royal Bank and mammoth holdings in utilities and paper, had special status. Holt exercised authority over $3 billion in corporate assets in 1928, when Canada only had $300 million in currency circulating, and hence, to some measurable extent, was the economy. He therefore could not help but feel the implosion acutely—but not personally. "Whatever else may have been the result of the Crash," his son once said, "I noted no change in my family's way of living."

Then there were those, such as Bernard Baruch in the United States, who were said to have made fortunes by selling short, those who had avoided the market altogether, and those who were said to have done this or that when in fact they had not. Médéric Martin, the former mayor of Montreal, kept hearing rumours that he had suffered a breakdown after losing $250,000 on Black Tuesday. He finally phoned the *Gazette* to report he was in perfect health and had never played the market at all, ever. On October 29, he said, he had been contentedly working in his garden at Laval-des-Rapides. And then there were even some people who saw the future clearly. Perhaps the first such statement by a Canadian came on October 30, when C. H. Carlisle, the president of Goodyear Tire and Rubber, implied strongly that the Crash, combined with the grain situation, made the country's economic outlook very bleak indeed.

Carlisle's words were as accurate as they were brave and level-headed. He was especially incisive in laying so much emphasis on wheat. The Canadian banks had lent out roughly $300 million on the current crop. Its failure to move meant that this money, representing nearly 25 per cent of all outstanding commercial loans, was frozen. More of the banks' money was tied up this way than in the stock market, though it was difficult to say which collapse—that of stocks or that of grain—had had the worse effect on lending institutions.

The banks had known, instinctively, logically, the way all aware professionals had known, that the day of retribution would be coming. Yet they could not stop giving call loans; to have done that would have wrecked things for sure. Instead, since about August 1929, they had been resisting any increase in the number of call loans and, at the same time, increasing the number of commercial loans (tight money permitting) to help shore up sagging business conditions. In fact, they were lending seven times more for business purposes than they were for stock market purposes when the Crash hit. But this still left them in a bad position. The value of securities, the collateral on which so much money had been borrowed, was now failing lower and lower. It would have been easy for the banks to panic, just as their customers were doing. But they did not, to their everlasting credit.

During the night of the 29th, when the brokerage house staffs were working late and the customers were understandably sleepless, a new wave of rumour broke, and this time the word was encouraging. Early indications were that, in Toronto at least, buying orders received since the close of the exchanges were up by as much as 50 per cent, while selling orders had fallen proportionately; this presaged a good day Wednesday. Word on the Rialto was also that the banks were making heavy calls on brokers with outstanding loans. Such stories as these would have wiped out the shaky post-Crash optimism had not the banks stepped in to say, correctly, that the stories were untrue. Here were the people actually in authority at the banks saying they were holding off; such statements were far better than even *good* rumours because they were true, because they were fact.

On Wednesday, the first such denial came from A. E. Phipps, the president of the Imperial and of the Canadian Bankers' Association. He was followed by Clarence Bogert of the Dominion and S. H. Logan of the Commerce. Soon still others joined in. Everyone knew that this measure was only a temporary expedient. But it was reassuring because it reflected confidence and good judgment at a time when those qualities were not much in evidence.

At about the same time as the banks acted, for instance, the federal finance minister, James A. Robb, publicly expressed fear for the future of the life insurance companies, so much of whose capital was tied up in the stock market. He allowed it to be inferred that he personally favoured legal restrictions on the amount of securities such companies could hold. As it happened, Robb only had a couple weeks to live. On November 13, exchanges across the country would observe five minutes of silence in his memory. It was to be the only quiet period in the markets that day: the 13th is when prices slipped once more after a fortnight of uneasy recovery.

The Crash created an echo that rang in the ears, and for a while people seemed a bit dizzy as they tried to gauge the true meaning of what had happened. The bad effects were immediate and widespread. A check of the steamship offices revealed that Canadians were moving en masse to cancel reservations on cruises to Europe and the West Indies. There was a run on small loan companies as people tried to get quick cash on their automobiles, and mortgage offices were swamped. Some cities, it was clear, were worse hit than others, though it was hard to find a logical pattern in their claims. Sudbury, for example, seemed to have had a disproportionately high percentage of speculators who had been in up to their necks, while Oshawa claimed not to be much affected.

There was no great faltering in business, though it was obvious that big corporations were caught off guard, if only to the extent that they had to modify their ambitions. In the States, Paramount and Warner Brothers announced that they would not merge as they had planned to do, and a three-way deal involving Kraft Cheese, Hershey Chocolate, and Colgate-Palmolive was also abandoned. In Canada, a merger was called off between Loblaws and Dominion Stores. There were also various legal consequences of the Crash. One Toronto speculator brought suit against his broker, claiming the firm had withheld securities rightfully his; on the same day, another Toronto broker sued a client, claiming breach of contract for the client's alleged failure to put up the margin he had agreed to. (In November, the New Brunswick Supreme Court set a precedent in ruling that verbal stock orders were binding.)

But as there were these and other signs of trouble, so were there reassurances. "Fundamentally sound" moved another giant step closer to cliché while leading capitalists, for their part, took what practical steps they could. In the States, U.S. Steel and American Can declared extra dividends, and Henry Ford announced he was cutting his prices. Henceforth, a touring car would be $440 (down $20), a standard coupe $500 (down $50), and a roadster $435 (down $15). John D. Rockefeller announced that stocks were good buys now that they were so cheap, and as the *Wall Street Journal* pointed out, "Only the foolhardy will combat John D.'s judgment." Later Rockefeller was more nearly emphatic: not only were some stocks good buys, he said, but his sons were purchasing in volume. And indeed it must be remembered, as Richard Sobel has pointed out, that 16 million shares sold in New York on Black Tuesday meant also that 16 million shares were *bought*. People with the necessary funds were suspected of preparing themselves for fire-sales. In time, there would be the stories of people becoming wealthy in this way, such as Floyd Odlum of Atlas Corporation, and Joe Kennedy. However, this was clearly not an option available to most of the people in the market in those first few weeks after Black Tuesday.

Wednesday, October 30, was a jittery day. A look-alike of Arthur Cutten created a great hubbub by innocently strolling onto the trading floor in Toronto. In New York, stocks rose markedly at first, but the momentum of the day before was bound to bring them back at least part way. At the close of trading, Richard Whitney appeared at the NYSE to announce that the exchange would be open only part of the day on Thursday and would remain closed until the following Monday. There were cheers. The people on the floor took this as an indication that the big bankers were going to shore up prices once again. But the exchange was closing only so that the backlog of work could be cleared up. In fact, the only reason the NYSE was open at all was to keep a "gutter market" from springing up in the streets of the financial district, as had been the custom in the old days.

For the first time in memory, the New York money markets stayed open Saturday when the NYSE was closed. Montreal and Toronto followed the New York lead on Thursday and opened at noon instead of at 10 a.m., though the Standard mining exchange kept its usual hours. But the two-hour delay didn't relieve all the confusion. The tickers were still far behind. International Nickel sold during the day for 40 in Europe but, owing to the poor communications, was quoted at 37½ in Toronto; one broker with a clear wire made a fat bankroll by buying locally and selling to London. Generally, in fact, the market behaved well that Thursday. Then came the long weekend crowded with good news and bad.

In the United States, several large corporations, including Bethlehem Steel, cancelled planned bond issues, and there were some bankruptcies announced. Yet even in the States the good seemed to outweigh the bad, and certainly this was the ratio in Canada as well. The Saturday *Star* in Toronto, noting that average industrials had now recovered about 70 per cent of Black Tuesday's level, was typical in its prognosis. "Basically, commerce has not been shaken; Canada's outlook continues to be a promising one," especially for people interested in long-term investment.

When brokerage workers in Montreal and Toronto went back to work on Monday, November 4, they found surprises in their pay packets. Grateful bosses had given many of them, in addition to a year-end bonus, an extra week's salary in recognition of the way they had been working uncomplainingly up to 24 hours at a stretch. As the day got officially under way, almost everyone looked forward to a rise in prices, what with the enforced cooling-off period. But then came the second surprise. The market once again failed to perform in the way expected, though no one could say precisely why this was the case.

In retrospect, it seems that closing down the markets was a mistake, for they were shut before prices could gravitate to whatever level the free market would have demanded. Shutting them down when they did, the *Mail and Empire* stated Monday, "was almost like halting a rugby match at its most heated point in order to allow the players a chance to recuperate." The holiday had, as intended, helped whittle down the paperwork, but even this had its negative side. The NYSE opened briskly and the ticker, with what was coming to seem its usual tardiness, was 28 minutes behind by 11 a.m. But then it caught up. At 1:37 p.m. it was actually up to the minute with prices for the first time since 11:17 a.m. on Wednesday, October 23, almost two full weeks earlier.

This sudden and not entirely expected sense of order brought out the bears. And this in turn brought out the bulls, a virgin crop of them from all indications. Some brokers reported 50 new customers that day, ones who had never speculated before.

> There are cases in Toronto [the *Mail and Empire* reported] where new investors bought Noranda, as one illustration, when it was under 30. On Saturday it sold at over 40 on the Standard exchange. A profit of thirty-three per cent in one week may very well go to their heads. With that repeated in thousands of cases all over Canada and the U.S., the problem of today's market becomes highly complicated.

A Toronto headline summed up the day most neatly: "MARKET UNDECIDED, SWINGS BOTH WAYS". This was not itself bad news, but it wasn't what had been expected. Once again the "marts" (as newspaper deskmen called them when faced with the problem of writing one-column heads) were moving by some power of their own. Yet the men in charge continued to decide in favour of short-er trading hours, so the pent-up energy had to be expended in that much briefer a time, with more dramatic effects.

Tuesday, November 5, for instance, the American markets re-mained closed because this was the date of the U.S. election. Montreal saw no point in opening by itself and so followed suit. But Toronto cockily remained open, only to see prices fall more than anyone had expected, wiping out the moderate gains of Monday. On Thursday the seventh, New York had decided, the close would be at 1 p.m. instead of 3 p.m.; once again Montreal and other cities fell into line but Toronto was determined to remain open all day. It changed its mind in the late morning, however. The markets on bal-ance rose. Then on Friday the eighth, another early-closing day, they fell again more or less across the board. Saturday all exchanges remained closed. It was Armistice Day, and veterans of the late war were out in force as early as 6 a.m. selling poppies. They told re-porters that more people than usual were putting coins in the collection boxes instead of folding money; they blamed the Crash. Monday the Montreal and Toronto exchanges were closed because it was Canadian Thanksgiving. New York remained open, of course, and recorded more of what was coming to be a pattern without de-sign: a rise, then a fall, followed by a more cautious rise and then a still greater fall.

Tuesday, the 12th of November, was the first day in a while, then, on which all the markets were opened at the same time and in approximately the same frame of mind. Even the Standard, which had been going its own bizarre way, conformed on the ques-tion of operating hours. There were heavy losses on the TSE; but for reasons no one could quite pinpoint, the MSE remained on a

relatively sound footing after recovering from the open jolt of selling. Then the next day, November 13, came the worst single bout
of trading since Black Tuesday.

The details begin to weary. Suffice to say another terribly grim
day was experienced on all fronts. This time it was more of the big
traders who were wiped out, not just the little and medium-sized
speculators. And this time the effects were almost instantly felt in the
retail economy. Orders for new cars, Persian rugs, houses, radios, pi-
anos, fur coats, and other luxury items were cancelled left and right,
and several large corporations began offering to lend money to employees who held company stock to keep these shares too from being
dumped. There hadn't yet been a run on savings accounts, at least not
in Canadian cities, but this might be coming. One Toronto broker
stated sadly that he had just lost a million dollars.

Even by the next day matters hadn't calmed down on the mi-
crocosmic environments of the stock exchange floors. R. E.
Knowles, the *Toronto Daily Star*'s hyperbolic feature-writer, looked
in on the TSE on Thursday morning. He found the scene "like a sort
of combination of a lion's cage at the zoo, a negro camp meeting of
1855, a riot in the Chicago Haymarket and a typhoon on the mid-
Pacific in the tropics." After that, prices continued to degenerate
but the newspapers lost interest. This particular form of bad news
had become old hat. The reality of the situation had become passé,
though, of course, this didn't make it less real.

Reaction to the events of November 13 was similar to what had followed Black Tuesday. The floors of the various exchanges were
littered not merely with paper but with the butts of thousands of
barely smoked cigarettes: an indication that the tension had been
running unusually high. There was the same sort of anonymous de-
spair there had been on October 30 and the same stories of
individual tragedy. Margaret Shotwell, a 19-year-old concert pi-
anist, lost the million dollars she had recently inherited from a
friend. A Toronto merchant, one "who did business on Yonge Street

so long that even to mention his line would instantly identify him," lost so much that he had to face seeking a job or borrowing from friends. The next few days, like those following the big collapse two weeks earlier, were also characterized by band-aid responses from the financial community, by a new generation of rumour, and by a good deal of hot air.

The heads of the Canadian banks, for instance, announced a reduction in margin requirements (their second in as many weeks) to 15 per cent on stocks selling over $30 and a flat $10 on those selling for more than that. This move brought what was now beginning to seem a knee-jerk response from brokerage people. To C. E. Abbs, the president of the Toronto Stock Exchange, it was a "helpful gesture by the bankers likely to fulfill its apparent intention of inspiring confidence among the public and of having a general reassuring effect." To the president of the Standard, Norman C. Urquhart, it was "one of the most constructive and reassuring moves ever made by the banks." He added: "The cool-headed businessmen of the country have, in effect, said they were satisfied the situation had gone too far. They are calling on the public to keep their heads and not sell their stocks below their real value." But it was difficult to be as coolheaded as these leaders were alleged to be, what with all the conflicting stories and the jumble of important and trivial information.

Those newspapers with a Protestant bias (that is to say, the entire English language press) sought to conceal their delight in rumours that the Vatican had been a heavy loser; the pontiff, it was said, had dropped a particularly large bundle in steel stocks. Closer to home, one Toronto broker was sued by Simpsons for a $1,056.60 clothing and cosmetics bill run up by his wife. A Toronto Transportation Commission driver found a ten-thousand-dollar bond on his Rosedale bus and returned it to the woman who'd presumably been on her way to cash it in. There were doom-sayers, as usual, and also those who looked on the bright side. R. E. Knowles met his match as master of vermilion prose in the magnate Sigmund

Samuel. "I should say that although happily we were not affected, yet comparatively few emerged unscathed," said Samuel. "I do not expect the present earthquake condition to continue. But even if it should, for a time, the ultimate result would not be altogether void of good. The experience, while bitter, is yet possessed of certain medicinal properties not to be despised."

In the ensuing weeks, however, it became clear that there was little reason for educated optimism, which is as good as saying that pessimism was entirely justified. The signs, official and otherwise, were there. In the States particularly a spate of embezzlements was discovered, the most scandalous involving the disappearance, from a bank in Flint, Michigan, of $3 million, which employees had frittered away on the market. Galbraith has suggested that this type of crime was a far more significant by-product of the Crash than suicide. On some days, short reports of embezzlements took up more than a column of the *New York Times* as a mood of suspicion took hold and surprise audits became common. A celebrated Canadian instance involved a 22-year-old employee of Canadian Oil Company who made off with twenty-nine thousand dollars of the firm's money and donated half of it to charity.

In Canada, many corporations, accustomed to issuing annual reports to lure investors, began producing instant mini-reports; the company out first with its information might be able to help stop its credibility from sagging. "Financial authorities and industrial heads," one columnist observed, "realize the job they have on their hands is to make the public believe the stock market reaction was healthy and in the best interests of all concerned and that there are no grounds for pessimism." But the propaganda wasn't going to work this time. "Stock market soothsayers have lost credit with the public and may have lost confidence in themselves," the *Montreal Star* said editorially on November 15. The forecasters persisted all the same. Three days later, for instance, Roger Babson, with remarkable gall, stated that unbeknownst to everyone a recession had actually begun last July.

In the middle of the month, the *Financial Post* reported on a private meeting of unnamed economists, statisticians, brokers, and bond dealers. They had met to compare notes on the U.S. situation and see what effect it might have on Canadian markets. "Young men who were optimists not long since have become extreme pessimists," the *Post* noted. "Older men who were pessimistic a few weeks ago are somewhat more optimistic." There was, in a phrase, a stalemate of opinion until later in the month when the consensus shifted in favour of the gloomy.

A. E. Phipps, the outgoing head of the Canadian Bankers' Association, told the group's annual meeting that the current situation would be followed by increased unemployment, a loss in purchasing power, and a general business decline. It was finally beginning to sink in that this time the stock market was not an autonomous playground but the mirror of an increasingly sick economy. Once the realization was articulated by a few people in authority it quickly spread and gained acceptance. In a few days, for instance, the *Financial Post* released the results of its seven-point assessment of business development for the year; the figures showed that a serious decline had been gathering momentum in Ontario, and this suggested the possibility of a recession in manufacturing all across the country. A concurrent turnabout was evident in the United States. Some New York brokerage house newsletters, which existed for the purpose of selling the future, now came out flatly and said the country's economy was going to the dogs.

At this point, the word being used in both countries was "recession", which suggests a short-term condition. But as the year came to a close the harsher noun, "depression", began cropping up here and there. Without a doubt, the transition from the 1920s to the 1930s was almost complete, not simply in the chronological sense but in the cultural terms that now distinguish the two decades in our common memory and imagination. Certain trappings and key images of the one age were being forgotten and others of the Depression era were gaining hold; sensibilities were changing. In mid-November, for instance, a group of New York society folk held a "poverty party" on Park Avenue. "With the stock market collapse as their inspiration," they arrived in old clothes (that is, last season's gowns), ate wieners and sauerkraut from tables covered with déclassé red cotton cloths, and stood around conversing by candlelight. In Canada, this did not at once catch on, though some of the University of Toronto students attending the annual Hart House masquerade did wear costumes that made comment on the Crash. Basically, though, the old ways lingered, with Sir Henry Pellatt's soirées at Casa Loma and Lady Eaton's galas at Ardwold. It was in other ways that the new order became apparent.

In 1928, for instance, a seat on the Montreal Stock Exchange had sold for $250,000. In September 1929 another went for a reputed $225,000. But in November the firm of Flood, Potter and Company made a bid of only $175,000. As it happened, the offer was rejected, but the precedent was set. No doubt about it, money was getting scarce and economizing was being practised at every level of society. The gardener at one of the gentlemen's clubs on Sherbrooke Street was instructed to stop using manure to protect outdoor plants against the snow; from now on he was to recycle the straw jackets then used on some champagne bottles.

In a remarkably short time, many people would be contemptuous of the very idea of champagne. They would feel, not entirely correctly, that the rich and the nouveaux riches had brought the world down into the Depression (for this is what it was now called) by their voracious appetite for stock-gambling. That the whole texture of society changed visibly, with relatively little overlapping of good and bad, can be shown in a hundred examples. One of the clearest, perhaps, is Vancouver, where cultural trends are often first visible.

In May 1929, the voters had approved a municipal bond issue worth almost $6 million; in December they voted for another one valued at $4.2 million. Such a public display of confidence in the future would probably have been impossible only a few weeks later. On December 17, a mob stormed the city relief office, set up in response to the growing population of people without jobs. Here the shadow recession, which had quietly worsened while the market boomed, was obvious. As early as 1925, the city had 10,000 white jobless and 3,500 out-of-work Chinese Canadians. Yet the building boom was getting under way and to all outward appearances the times were good as almost never before. One Vancouver peculiarity was a penchant for huge, garish electric signs, including a three-storey bottle of beer spilling its neon contents into a glass almost as large. Now these trappings of success seemed to mock the people at the bottom end of the economic scale, the ones who were first to feel the shock waves.

On December 18, several hundreds of them marched. The city responded with a ban on any further such demonstrations. Matters simmered a while longer. On the last day but one of 1929, the unemployed, now up 300 per cent in number, finally clashed with police. Many were arrested. The authorities spoke of how the city was being threatened by this "red army". It wasn't an army and it wasn't red but it continued growing, as refugees from the East poured into Vancouver to be spared at least the discomfort of snow. By the fall of 1930 there were 7,000 men on relief in Vancouver and hobo jungles were assuming shape under bridges and viaducts; one breadline contained more than 1,200 people.

Elsewhere in the country the details differed considerably but the tenor was the same. The Great Depression was all too seriously under way, with no end in sight; the gold digger, in the fiduciary and co-educational sense of the word, was already obsolete and forgotten.

10

Surviving the Thirties

It is almost irresistibly tempting to assess the story of the Crash in terms of individual human lives. Such illustrations simplify the complex aftermath and often have an ironic appeal. As a result of the Crash, for instance, John M. Millar and his wife Anne were forced to leave Winnipeg and move to the United States. Although their 14-year-old son Kenneth would return to Canada for a time, the move set in motion his affinity for a certain American lifestyle. It was a fascination he has put to good use, under the pseudonym Ross Macdonald, in creating the Lew Archer detective novels that so accurately depict the underside of Southern California.

But tales of hardship (and some of them are very graphic indeed) seldom do justice to the breadth of the problem the way a straightforward recital of some statistics can do. By 1933 some 15 per cent of the population, or about 1.5 million people, were receiving unemployment or drought relief. This figure would increase by another 500,000 the following year before starting to recede slowly—so slowly in fact that by 1938 there were still about 845,000 people on the pogey.

There was considerable variance in the percentage on relief from one community to the next, just as there were often different programs to cope with the problem in each area. Company towns were particularly hard hit, for instance, as were those in whose industries a slump was becoming obvious even before the Crash. In early 1932, for instance, the relief rate was 7.3 per cent in Kitchener, Ontario, with its farming and secondary manufacturing, but 38.6 per cent 185 miles away in East Windsor, with its heavy dependence upon the automotive industry. In some places the rate shot up as much as 1,000 per cent in a two-year period, and hundreds of small municipalities (particularly on the Prairies) went into default, only to be bailed out ultimately by Ottawa. Columns of figures, however, are not much use in showing the social and pyschological harm done in this period. And relying on them tends to meld rather than separate the two overlapping ideas, the Crash and the Depression.

One historian, Michiel Horn, has assessed the effects of the Depression upon the three identifiable sectors of the economy at the time, the farming class and the working class, totalling about 80 per cent of the country, and the amorphous middle classes, who made up most of the remaining 20 per cent. These last tended to be urban people, though many were the children of farmers, and their annual income ranged from $1,500 to a maximum of $10,000 a year. They were professionals, clerical workers, managerial and commercial people, and small businessmen. The farmers and the workers represent the Depression in our imaginations, Horn claims, though possibly the middle class were more important to the historical scheme of things. "They suffered much less from unemployment than the working class, but they had also been much less used to it before the Depression." This was where the change was most pronounced. Certainly it was here, and not in the factories or the fields, that the Crash was significant as a self-contained event.

Horn extrapolates from his own interpretation of American statistics that perhaps only 2 or 3 per cent of Canadians owned non-interest-bearing securities during the long boom. The figure seems conservative. But even if correct it still makes for a considerable impact on the middle classes: the 2 or 3 per cent, by his reckoning, could constitute up to 10 per cent of the under-$10,000 middle class—that is, aside from the rich people, who were a definite minority. In 1929, for instance, only 13,447 Canadians declared taxable income of more than $10,000 and this was down to 6,440 in 1934.

Figures like these make the amounts lost in the Crash and its various after-shocks all the more impressive. To state that the paper valuation of a short list of key Canadian stocks went down by a million dollars a minute is still quite a frightening fact. But inflation has deprived us of a sense of just how large a sum that was 50 years ago. If tax returns, once again, are a reliable indication, there were only some six hundred millionaires in the entire United States in 1929; today probably three hundred Americans have become millionaires just by holding McDonald's hamburger franchises. It was a different world, conducted on a different scale. Only the relative number of poor people in Canada has remained more or less unchanged since the Depression.

Although it's seldom considered in such discussions, the securities business itself must surely have been one of the hardest-hit fields. Here again, though, there were regional differences. Although many were insolvent, no member firm of the Toronto Stock Exchange actually went bankrupt in the years immediately following the Crash. And A. E. Ames, at least in legend, was the only brokerage house to come through the Depression unscathed. On the Montreal Stock Exchange, by contrast, bankruptcies were frequent for a time. On October 5 and 6, 1931, four companies were suspended because they were unable to meet their commitments. The first of the batch to go belly up was MacDougall and Cowans, which had been possibly the biggest brokerage firm in Canada at one time. It was so busy immediately before the Crash that it took the unprecedented step of refusing any more customers; its back shop was literally working 24 hours a day.

In brokerage as in other businesses, it was a time of personal sacrifice and sometimes a kind of heroism, too. There is a story that

Arthur Nesbitt, of Nesbitt Thomson, refused to cut the salaries of his workers and made up the difference out of his own pocket. And there was an instance of employees banding together to save one Vancouver firm, Burke, Smith and Marrow. The story comes from Bill Borrie, who joined the firm in 1925.

> One afternoon in 1931, Stanley Burke [the father of the broad-caster] called several senior salesmen into his office to announce that the bond department was broke and that a notice of closure would appear on the locked door at 411 Howe Street in the morning. The Bank of Commerce had accepted our collateral in the morning but rejected it in the afternoon and called an outstanding $80,000 loan. The collateral was mostly pulp and paper issues which were part of our inventory as agents of Wood Gundy.
>
> We had no capital to stave off the trouble, but the salesmen thought they could scrounge enough to stay in, if the partners would agree. After a long meeting it was decided to postpone the closing and meet again in the morning. The seniors decided they would raise or guarantee enough to pacify the bank. They held a session with the partners, who agreed to retain a minimal interest and sell the balance to the senior salesmen. So the Royal Bank was approached. They, being Wood Gundy's bankers and probably loaded with similar securities, agreed to accept our collateral guarantees, pay off the Commerce, and give us limited working capital.

It was not entirely a time of faltering business, however. After the Crash bankruptcies skyrocketed, but it's worth remembering that neither in number nor in dollar terms did they equal the business failures in the recession after the First World War. People hung on as best they could, and many persons still young enough not to be totally dispirited actually started up in business. In 1930, "Wacky" Bennett opened a hardware store in Kelowna, B.C. In

1931, Roy Thomson initiated what became his international communications empire by setting up a one-horse radio station in North Bay. In 1932, there was Charlie Burns. Later a partner of E. P. Taylor and the chairman of Crown Life, he was known only as the son of the president of the Bank of Nova Scotia when he borrowed $500 and established the Burns Brothers investment house, which was a particularly shrewd move. U.S. securities were often more undervalued than Canadian ones, and there were bargains in bonds and debentures on both sides of the border. As times eased up, and the economy reached a recessionary plateau of sorts, an eager broker could do well patching up damaged portfolios. This was especially true, as Burns must have foreseen, in Toronto.

If there was one instance of the Crash, as distinct from the rest of the Depression, being important in itself, it was the expediting of the rise of Toronto over Montreal as a financial centre. The fact that all of Toronto's brokerage houses survived is one indication of this. Another factor is the way the Toronto-based mining industry continued to flourish, if only in fits and starts. But a third consideration is that Toronto's stock market began to bound ahead of Montreal's once it cleaned itself up and once both of them lost at least a bit of their slavish dependence upon New York.

In September 1931, the British abandoned the gold standard to which Churchill had returned them only a few years earlier. All imperial currencies were immediately hurt; the Canadian dollar was discounted 25 per cent in New York. The market became so demoralized that the Toronto exchanges pegged prices, feeling that otherwise the numbers would not reflect market values fairly. This was not itself, of course, a good time for the Canadian exchanges. But it did show the TSE and the Standard working together as one and did indicate action independent of the rest of the world. Then in March 1933 Roosevelt declared his moratorium on banking (causing the U.S. dollar to fall 35 cents overnight in Canada). In every state banks were shut down; the Chicago Board of Trade was closed for the first time in 85 years; and the U.S. stock exchanges suspended activity for two weeks. The Canadian exchanges kept going, however, just as they would do during the Second World War, and it was to Toronto and not to Montreal that people usually looked to get some indication of the value of their American securities.

But 1934 was the cincher. In January, Roosevelt made his decision to fix gold at $35. This stimulated prices in Toronto for three or four years to come. Meanwhile, in February, the Toronto Stock Exchange and the Standard finally merged, to the relief of many in all areas of business and all political parties. The two remained in separate buildings, however, until construction of the present Ticker Palace (as the *Star Weekly* called it) was completed in 1937, at a cost of $750,000, or about the same amount the exchange would pay for a single computer in the 1960s.

By now, there was no question of Toronto's being the first financial city of Canada even if it lagged behind in population and in other ways. The TSE now not only outstripped the MSE in dollar volume but exceeded the New York Curb in share volume, and so was second in this regard only to the NYSE. When the building opened, the new exchange was the subject of a major story in *Time*. Its chairman, Harry Broughton, was the first Canadian businessman on the cover of that magazine, which had not yet begun its controversial Canadian edition and dealt only with such passing Canadian subjects as Mary Pickford and the Dionne quints. "Politically, financial Toronto is about as liberal as the Archbishop of Canterbury," *Time* commented, "but in spirit the Liberal Government of Prime Minister King is close to exciting Toronto, just as the previous Conservative Government of pious Richard Bedford Bennett was close to decorous Montreal." The point was well taken. The emphasis had indeed shifted and with it the tone of Canadian financial dealings. Toronto finance assumed a style different from that of Montreal finance. The stock market was an important indication of this, perhaps the single most significant one, in fact. But for all that, the market, as always, was only a reflection of a larger reality.

Toronto was now fast becoming the business centre of the country's anglophone population. It matched Montreal in some areas and began getting ahead in others. Montreal, for instance, had long had the Canadian Pacific, but Toronto became more important in its own right after creation of the Canadian National. Then there were the huge national retailing concerns, such as Eaton's and Simpsons, to say nothing of the important manufacturing corporations and various other head offices. Also, of course, there was the legitimate opening of the northland by the major mining firms. Even Noranda, though located in north-eastern Quebec, got its major push from Toronto. But as long as mining still played an important role in the Toronto securities business there would always, it seemed, be a low element giving the city a bad name. In time, however, even the charlatans, the last reminder of the free-wheeling bull market days, were weeded out.

No sooner had the good times returned, at the end of the Second World War, than Toronto was again full of bucket shops and boiler-rooms, terms that were by now becoming interchangeable. This new wave of fraudulent activity had a lot to do with the expansion of mining to include vanadium, niobium, and especially uranium, though the renewed upward trend of the economy was the main factor. As before, many of the sharp operators were Americans, including one notorious fellow who made $4,000 a week peddling securities in Canada even though he had jumped a $50,000 bail in the States. And once again, many of the suckers were Canadians who should have known better. But in the main, this new outcropping of chicanery consisted of Canadians selling stocks in non-productive, even non-existent, mines to American residents, usually by telephone or through the mails.

The American authorities were understandably upset. A 1951 report of the U.S. Securities and Exchange Commission spoke of "these greedy, ruthless men [who] have been milking gullible Americans from Toronto for years ...." The SEC put the total take at $52 million a year and tried to get the Ontario government to crack down. The Ontario

Securities Commission replied that it estimated the lucre at only $9 million. Besides, some internal policing was already being done.

In 1947, the Broker-Dealer Association began, with almost two hundred members, to get rid of the bounders before the OSC could indeed come down hard. But the crooked operations were too large, and the loopholes too numerous, for any such watchdog group to be totally effective. Finally, the SEC persuaded the American postal authorities to refuse to handle the direct-mail pieces of the Ontario promoters. Later, in 1961, the dealers themselves banned across-the-border selling.

Other provinces, notably British Columbia and Quebec, would clean up their own securities rackets to a remarkable degree. But most of the emphasis was still on Ontario: a further proof that that is where the action was. With the bucketeers gone, some attention focused on the legitimate members of the TSE, particularly the stringency of membership requirements and the alleged conflict of interest that arose when brokers traded too advantageously on their own accounts as well as on their customers'. There were several inquiries and royal commissions, and various good works in the field were instigated by the legislature. One of the figures prominent in such matters was Kelso Roberts, the provincial attorney general.

Roberts, in a privately published autobiography, got at what he considered the one remaining bugaboo in the system: gossip. "Unfortunately in the trading practices of today," he wrote, "once a rumour is circulated it can very quickly lose the characteristics of rumour and become acceptable as fact. Therein lies the great danger." Certainly this was the case in the late 1920s, though there was another even more important intangible at work in the wildest bull market ever known. There was a faith (misplaced, as it happened) in the future. All else being equal, it is that optimism, rooted not just in the greed of gold diggers but in the existence of a far less complex and threatening world, that allowed the events of 1929 to get out of control. Such faith, it seems, can never recur, and this perhaps is the saddest fact about Canada and the great Crash.

Epilogue

Can it happen again? Ah, there's the question. But the answers (for there are several important variations on the simple Yes and No) must each be seen in terms of another set of uncertainties. For instance, what really caused the Crash of 1929? What would be necessary to bring about a similar set of conditions today? And how could another crash on the 1929 scale take place even without those exact same stimuli? Such matters can (and frequently do) fill books far larger than this narrative.

One obvious consideration is that while the 1929 debacle was *the* Crash, it was by absolutely no means the first, last, or only. One could go back to the bursting of the South Sea Bubble in the 18th century and still deal with the subject in terms of its similarities to the modern age, even though crashes have seldom had many of the same tangible components. In 1922, one economic historian drew up a long list of what people had supposed to be the causes of various past calamities of this kind. The list included public and personal stinginess, public and personal extravagance, excessive gold imports, excessive gold exports, the inflation of currency, the deflation of currency, the failure of women to get the vote, the rise in telegraph rates, the custom of free railway passes, the use of to-bacco, and, of course, sunspots.

Today this cumulative litany has undergone a considerable shakedown, and the process continues. No one now seriously be-lieves, for instance, what many took as gospel a half-century ago: that the Crash was largely the fault of a few fat cats manipulating Wall Street. But there is still some debate on what were the base causes—over and above the obvious elements, such as uninformed mass speculation through the use of leverage and margin, and the cultural climate that encouraged it.

To some extent the range of opinion can almost be broken down along political lines. Economics resembles psychology in being not-quite-a-science, and, moreover, a quite factionalized one. Just as the Freudians differ with the Jungians, and they both dis-agree with the Gestalt people, so Keynesians are at odds with the monetarists, and together they all fail to get along with moderates, who seem so unextreme as to be almost without conviction. Generally speaking, the doom-sayers would appear to have the greater claim on public attention, regardless of whether they exer-cise a forensic advantage.

A big segment of the society would seem to *want* to believe that a great cataclysmic economic crash is imminent because the world (as difficult as this is to believe) has grown too bland for them. Purveyors are happy to oblige, for optimism is not what brings large paperback advances and sells overpriced newsletters. Yet the pet scenario of such people is not precisely a replay of 1929, though it would have the same effects or worse. They see the cause for alarm as being the undeniably real danger of runaway inflation re-sulting in social instability, not simply excessive speculation.

This is where the political and the economic become one. At one time it was thought that inflation came only from governments printing too much money and that the free-market system would eventually achieve full employment. But Keynes turned these no-tions upside down. He saw inflation as partly the result of struggles between various economic classes and believed unemployment was inevitable without government policy to keep it down; in fact, he felt recessions were part of long series of disequilibria caused by the lack of effective controls.

He was the litmus. Those who came after him either agreed with the principles and translated them for use in current situations or harked back to a far simpler view. In the former category one finds, for instance, Galbraith. The latter includes the monetarists and the extreme right wing. It encompasses people who still think inflation is just the result of too much paper money and those who want to return to the gold standard. Or those who see a cycle of boom and depression caused by government interference in the economy, and those to whom inflation is simply postponing the next big depression and making the prospect more horrible.

There's no mistaking it: the whole question is tied up with political squabbling and uncertainty as it never was in 1929. This is not to single out party politics necessarily but rather the System, the feeling that only governments can get us into trouble and only governments can get us out again. It's a state of mind that encourages paranoia in some and a sense of impermanent comfort in others.

There are those who feel that the powers that be (Them) have secretly committed us to a policy of periodic mini-depressions. This is similar to the view held in more liberal sections of the Pentagon about an endless series of limited, brushfire wars instead of the one final blast. These are the people who believe that ideas derived from Keynes (various kinds of government policy and control), though they may have been the solution to the last depression, will be the cause of the next. Then again there are those who feel, what with the very considerable imponderables of inflation, petro-economics, Third World realignment, and the threat of nuclear war, that the financial system itself is a little island of relative strength because of its institutionalized flexibility.

Given all that, what can one say about the stock market itself and the Canadian market particularly? It seems safe to make at least one generalization: to the extent (mainly psychological) that the Crash *was* the cause of the Depression, the reverse would probably be the case in the future, with the collapse of the market a consequence of some greater upheaval in the society at large. The market is almost as tightly controlled today as the whole economy, and for this and other reasons not so susceptible to wildcat speculation. A crash, after all, is nothing but a too-fast economic slowdown, just as an explosion is a too-fast burning of fuel; and to have a crash you must first have a market boom, and these have been infrequent. In 1962, for instance, there was a bad slide, but this was caused mainly by outside political developments in the United States. Then there was the recession of 1973–74, attributable largely to political events of even broader significance. Between them there was only one giant wave of speculative fever, resulting in the market crash of 1969–70.

Other factors aside, any bull market remotely like that of the 1920s would be as dissimilar as it would be similar. For one thing, markets outside this continent—Tokyo's, for example—are more important than ever before. But even without that redress of financial power, Wall Street is changing. Electronics are making some of its dynamic obsolescent. So is the drift of financial power from New York to Washington, D.C. Fiscal power in Canada is shifting also, and the first stage is already complete; the Montreal Stock Exchange is scarcely more than a shell, with the organization itself recording sizeable deficits in some years.

So there is, then, something to be said for both the negative and the affirmative points of view. Nations are much more interdependent than they were 50 years ago but face collective problems not foreseeable back then. And it's probably wise to remember that in 1929 the economic woods were full of people, many of them leading business thinkers of the time, who thought a crash on the scale of 1920-21 impossible.

Given as nearly the same set of circumstances as possible, Canada would doubtless perform better today than it did in the Crash and the Great Depression. We are still saddled with many of the old problems: an abundance of company towns, for instance, and a general lack of economy diversification on the Prairies. But the economic structure can better withstand economic shocks of the kind felt in the 1930s, when the government had little or no experience in using fiscal and monetary tools to adjust imbalances and lacked the kind of social-welfare schemes we now take for granted. And Canadians these days invest far more in their own country than their fathers or grandfathers did. What's more, Canadian manufacturing has grown up considerably, though this sector is still foreign-dominated. For the record, however, Galbraith distinguishes between the threat of foreign ownership in such a situation and "the massive intertwining of the two economies" generally. "But given a recession of the sort one had in the 1930s or milder," he admits, "the effects on Canada would be indistinguishable from those in the United States."

Galbraith himself is perhaps a good place to end the discussion, as his prominence in the field of economics has made him a sort of unwilling touchstone for the type of hypersensitivity one sees in glancing backward to 1929. In 1955, he appeared before the Banking and Currency Committee of the U.S. Senate and testified that the stock market appeared to be begging for a crash some time in the future. The press gave his testimony exaggerated coverage, and this brought on a short-lived panic. He was roundly condemned for arousing pessimism, and one senator even accused him of communist inclinations (such was the custom then). There was also backlash after he made a similar prediction in 1960.

Then, in 1969, Galbraith was in Los Angeles on a political errand and was asked by reporters if another big crash was likely. This was at a time when speculation was indeed prevalent and widespread, and Galbraith answered offhandedly that of course another crash would come, the only question was when. Once again the story was given big play. Once again he was damned (and in some quarters praised) for putting the country on standby panic. From that point on he became more cautious in his wording. "What is necessary for a new disaster," he wrote in an article for *Harper's*, "is only for memories of the last one to fade and no one knows how long that takes."

So, finally, only history can judge whether 1929 will seem more important in the future than it did at the time, whether it was a significant event in itself or only the loudest in a series of warnings.

Sources and Acknowledgements

Most of what has been written on the Crash of 1929 deals with events in the United States. This literature is fairly extensive but is dominated by a few famous works. The best known, perhaps, is *The Great Crash, 1929* (Houghton Mifflin, 1955) by John Kenneth Galbraith, who synopsizes the basic ideas therein in several subsequent books, such as *The Age of Uncertainty* (Houghton Mifflin, 1977). Like nearly all the latterday Crash analysts, Galbraith drew to some extent on Frederick Lewis Allen's *Only Yesterday* (Harper, 1931), which despite (or because of) its closeness to the times has remained a remarkably useful look at American politics and culture in the 1920s.

Anyone interested in Wall Street lore should also examine the writings of Robert Sobel. The most specific in this case is *The Great Bull Market: Wall Street in the 1920s* (Norton, 1968). But others of interest are *Panic on Wall Street: A History of American Financial Disasters* (Macmillan, 1968), *N.Y.S.E.: A History of the New York Stock Exchange 1935-1975* (Weybright and Talley, 1975), and *Inside Wall Street* (Norton, 1977). Some are more pertinent to the Crash than others but they're all informed with a rare combination of the journalist's know-how and the historian's care. Sobel's bibliographies are often a joy in themselves.

A more recent work, which treats October 24 as an unfolding drama, is *The Day America Crashed* by Tom Shachtman (Putnam, 1979). Then there are the memoirs of those who participated in the actual events, including curiosities such as Roger Babson's autobiography, *Actions and Reactions* (Harper, 1935; later revisions). There also exist several books dealing with America as a whole in that *anno mirabilis* 1929; the best of these is *What a Year!* (Harper, 1956) by the late Joe Alex Morris, who was martyred in Iran while the present book was getting under way. In addition, of course, there are many studies of the Depression, both popular and scholarly, which take the Crash as their starting point. Among the most convenient is *The Great Depression: The United States in the Thirties* by Robert Goldston (Bobbs-Merrill, 1968).

In recent years, Canada has also had many books on the Depression. One I found especially useful was *The Dirty Thirties: Canadians in the Great Depression*, an anthology of documents edited by Michiel Horn (Copp Clark, 1972). Aside from these, most books touching on the Crash in Canada are serious economic studies, works of regional history, or biographies and autobiographies.

In the first category, the standard reference is A. E. Safarian's *The Canadian Economy in the Great Depression* (University of Toronto Press, 1959; Carleton Library, 1970) which is not surpassed for statistical evidence of Canada's economic rigidity and the slowness of its recovery. But one foreign study, *The World in Depression 1929-1939* (Allen Lane The Penguin Press, 1973), by the prolific economist Charles P. Kindleberger, is a useful appendix to Safarian in that it shows Canada in an international context. Also valuable are three other standard works: *An Economic History of Canada* by Mary Quayle Innis (Ryerson, 1935; revised 1943), *Chartered Banking in Canada* by A. B. Jamieson (Ryerson, 1953; later revisions), and *The Financial System of Canada: Its Growth and Development* by E. P. Neufeld (Macmillan of Canada, 1972).

The Prairies are the area best served by regional and local histories, and among the most useful and popular works are those of James H. Gray. Three of them deal with the destruction of the grain market and the boom in Western mining and oil: *The Winter Years* (1966), *The Roar of the Twenties* (1975), and Gray's autobiography, *Troublemaker!* (1978). All are published by Macmillan of Canada. *A Short History of Prairie Agriculture* by H. G. L. Strange (Searle Grain Co., Winnipeg, 1954) contains data on yearly crop yields and the like. Others I found helpful were *Tides in the West* by Leonard D. Nesbitt (Modern Press, Saskatoon, n.d.), a history of the Alberta Wheat Pool; and *Henry Wise Wood of Alberta* (University of Toronto Press, 1950), a life of the head of the United Farmers of Alberta by his brother, William Kirby Wood. Then, in addition to these works on the Prairie provinces, there are histories of individual Canadian cities. The ones that seemed to me most concerned with the Crash and the events immediately following it include: *The Story of Toronto* by G. P. deT. Glazebrook (University of Toronto Press, 1971), *Montreal: A Brief History* by John Irwin Cooper (McGill-Queen's University Press, 1969), and *Vancouver* by Eric Nicol (Doubleday Canada, 1970; revised 1978).

Biographical studies I have drawn on are *J. E. Atkinson of the Star* by Ross Harkness (University of Toronto Press, 1963), a life of the Toronto publisher Holy Joe Atkinson; *Louis St. Laurent: Canadian* by Dale C. Thomson (Macmillan of Canada, 1967); and *Flame of Power* by Peter C. Newman (Longman Canada, 1959). Especially well suited to my purpose was *A Gentleman of the Press* (Doubleday Canada, 1969), a biography of the magazine publisher Colonel John B. Maclean by his protégé, Floyd S. Chalmers.

Most of the information in the present book, however, was gleaned from accounts in those newspapers mentioned in the text. I have also drawn, however, on later articles about the Crash. These are "The Day a Whole Generation Went Broke" by John Gray (*Maclean's*, October 15, 1954), "The '29 Crash: Could It Happen Again" by Alexander Ross (*Maclean's*, November 1969), and "How

Stocks Crumbled 40 Years Ago" by Douglas Watt (the *Financial Post*, November 1, 1969). Michiel Horn's article "The Great Depression: Past and Present" (*Journal of Canadian Studies*, February 1976) contains useful figures on unemployment, relief, and similar matters; and "When Boiler Rooms Were In Bloom" by William Stephenson (*Financial Post Magazine*, May 1979) is a lively description of the post-Second World War mining cons on Bay Street.

Thanks are also due those witnesses who are quoted in the text, as well as many authors who elaborated upon their writing for me and otherwise provided information. Among the latter were John Kenneth Galbraith and A. E. Safarian. Persons who are both firsthand observers as well as authors are Floyd S. Chalmers, who graciously allowed me access to his unpublished memoirs, and James H. Gray, who shared his knowledge of the wheat fiasco.

Also helpful were Susan Baptie of the Vancouver City Archives, the City of Toronto Archives, Alastair Dow, the Montreal Stock Exchange, Barry Morgan, Blair Neatby, the Toronto Public Libraries, particularly the Yorkville and central reference branches, the Toronto Stock Exchange, and Anne Marie Uppal of the Canadian Imperial Bank of Commerce. Finally my thanks to Roger Hall of the University of Western Ontario and Michiel Horn of York University, who read and criticized the manuscript. Errors of fact and interpretation, however, are of course my own.

Appendices

Quotations from the Toronto Stock Exchange, Tuesday, October 29, 1929

1929 High	Low	Stocks	Sales	Open	High	Low	Cl'se	Net Ch'ge
20	4⅛	Asbestos, new . . .	50	4⅛	. . .	. . .	. . .	– ¼
60	41½	B.C. Pow., "A" . .	50	41½	. . .	. . .	. . .	– 2⅞
40	23½	Do., "B"	40	23½	. . .	. . .	. . .	– 4½
182	154	Bell Tele., ...	199	158	159	154	156	– 4
10.00	3.75	Bell rts.	295	5.00	5.00	3.75	4.00	– 1.00
82	40½	Brazilian, n.	15,315	49	49	40½	43	– 8
46	25	Bldg. Prod., c. . .	290	28	28	25	25½	– 4
90	45	Burt. F., c.	202	49	49	45	45	– 11
122	108⅞	Can. Bread p. A. .	5	118½	. . .	. . .	. . .	+ ½
28½	20	Do., new	1,206	21	21	20	21	unch
37	9	Can. Brewing . . .	15	10	10	9	9	– 1
28	17	C. Canners, c. . .	565	19½	20	17	17½	– 3
95	87½	Do. 1st pfd. . . .	214	88¼	89	87½	87½	– 1½
28	18	Do. 2nd pfd. . . .	. . .	20¾	21	18	18	– 3
29½	19⅝	Can. Car new . . .	335	19¾	20¼	19⅝	19⅝	– 4⅝
. . .	. . .	Do., pref.	600	25¼	. . .	. . .	. . .	. . .
36	19	Can. Cemt. c. . . .	90	20	20	19	19	– 1½
99	91¼	Do., pref.	45	93	94½	93	93	– 3
89¾	33	Can. Dredg. c. . .	983	37	39	33	36	– 4
97	64	Can. Dry	25	64	. . .	. . .	. . .	– 12½
32⅞	20½	C. Gypsum-Al . .	975	24	24	20½	23	– 2
60½	57	C. Gen. Ele. p. . .	10	58	. . .	. . .	. . .	+ ½
47	8	C. Ind. Alcoh. . . .	385	12	12	8	11	– 1
75	35	Can. Oil, new . . .	45	40	40	35	35	– 8
265	195	C.P.R.	37	198	200	195	195	– 15
97¾	76⅜	C. S.S.L., pfd. . .	20	76⅜	. . .	. . .	. . .	– 2⅛
89	35	C. Dairy, c.	935	45	49	35	47	– 5

1929 High	Low	Stocks	Sales	Open	High	Low	Cl'se	Net Ch'ge
52¼	17½	Cockshutt	885	24	26	17½	20	– 5
24	16	Conduits, n.	70	16½	16½	16	16	– ¾
43	18	Consol. Bak.	7,692	25	25	18	20	– 5
196	184¼	Cons. Gas	298	187	187½	186	186	– 1½
29⅞	18	Cosmos Imp. c. ..	370	19	19	18	18	– 2
161	95½	Do., pref.	5	98	...	...	...	– 1
9	3½	Duluth Sup.	50	3½	...	...	...	– ½
53	32	East'n St. P.c.. ..	165	36	...	...	...	– 4
40	15	E. Washing. M. ..	25	17	17	15	15	– 1
81½	34½	Fam. Play.	35	49	52	46	46	– 5
70	23	Ford. Mtr. "A" ...	4,200	30	30	23	25	– 9¼
15	14	Fr-Wire, c.	20	15	15	14½	14½	unch
98	93	Do., pref.	25	94	95	94	95	+ 1
40	22	G.S. Wares	378	25	25	22	24	– 4
110½	106	Goodyear, p.	360	107	107	106½	106½	– 1
32	5	G.W. Sadd., c. ..	340	5	...	...	...	unch
35½	25	H. Cottons, p. ..	40	25	...	...	...	unch
11	4	Ham. U. Th., c. .	140	5	...	...	...	– 1½
65	35	Hayes Wh., c. ...	45	35	...	...	...	– 10
165	100	Do., pref.	20	101	...	...	...	unch
57	39	L. Secord	770	50	51	46	46	– 8
24½	9	Loblaw, "B"	615	9	10	9	10	– 3
24½	9	Do., "A"	1,835	13	13	9	10	– 3
35	25	M. Leaf, c.	50	28	...	...	...	– 2
115	105	Do., pref.	15	108	109	108	109	– 1
98¾	35	M. Harris, c. ...	3,350	39	40	35	39	– ½
36½	22	Moore, c.	665	26½	28	22	23	– 5
141	120	Do., "A" pfd. ...	5	120	...	...	...	unch
106	100	N. Grocers, p. ..	35	103	...	...	...	unch
70	35	Ont. Eq. Life ...	15	35	...	...	...	– 12
97¾	65	Orange C. 1st p. .	5	65	...	...	...	unch
140	78	Page-Hersey	3,005	95	100	78	84	– 16
45	23	Photo Eng.	595	26½	26½	23	24½	– 1½
43	19½	Pressed Met. n. ..	290	31	31⅛	28	28½	– 2½
40	20	Pure Gold	50	25	...	...	...	unch
26	16	Quality Can. ...	50	16	...	...	...	– 4
26	21	Riverside S.A. ..	125	21	21	20	20	– 4
105	91	Simpson's p.	154	92	92	91	91½	– ½
45	33	Do., B.	33	38	38	36	36	– 3
20	12	Stan. Stl. c.	15	12	...	...	...	unch
48	37	Do., pfd.	5	43	...	...	...	+ ½
69	39	Steel of Can. c. ..	255	55	55	39	39	– 12
48½	37	Tip Top T. c.	290	42	42	40	40	– 2½
113	105	Do. pfd.	25	105	...	...	...	unch
28½	8	Walker's G.-W. ..	34,543	10¼	10½	8	9¼	– 1¾
115	25	Weston Ltd. c. ..	25	25	...	...	...	– 17
108	55	Win. Elec. c. ...	100	55	...	...	...	– 1¼
		Mines—						
570	270	Cons. Smelt. ...	41	300	300	270	270	– 50
72¼	29	Int. Nickel Cn. ..	109,530	35	37	29	32½	– 6¼

1929

High	Low	Stocks	Sales	Open	High	Low	Cl'se	Net Ch'ge
27.00	18.00	Lake Shore	100	18.00	...	...	...	− 2.10
		Banks—						
360	272	Commerce	66	275	285	272	275	− 10
280	240	Dominion	88	241	245	240	240	− 2
275¼	245	Imperial	186	250	252¼	245	248	− 4
417	321¼	Montreal	5	340	...	...	...	unch
395	320	Royal	130	328	332	320	320	− 14
281½	250	Toronto	25	264	...	...	...	− 3¾
		Loan, Trust, Etc.—						
105	98	Can. Gen. Inv.	15	100	...	...	...	unch
280	250	Tor. Gen. T.	10	250	...	...	...	unch

UNLISTED

High	Low	Stocks	Sales	Open	High	Low	Cl'se	Net Ch'ge
27½	20	Beath and Son	5	21	...	...	...	− 3
59	30	Beatty Bros., c.	1,035	40	40	30	30	− 11
49⅛	30	Bissell com.	40	32	...	...	...	+ 2
150	98	Do., pfd.	47	98	...	...	...	unch
71¼	39	B.A. Oil	29,071	46	46	39	39⅛	− 11½
12	7	Can. Bud. Brew	120	9⅛	9½	7⅛	7½	− 2
35	10	Can. Malt.	1,425	16½	17	11	15	− 2
41	25	Can. Pav. com	5	28	...	...	...	unch
132⅛	93	Do., pfd.	90	97	97	93	93	− 4
42¼	29	Can.Vinegar	575	30	30	29	29	− 4
27	18	Can. Wire Box	470	18	19	18	18½	− ¼
35½	4½	Carling's	535	5	5½	4½	5	unch
12¾	7	Crown Dom. Oil	10	8	...	...	...	− ½
21	14½	De Forest	110	17	17	14½	14½	− 3½
25¾	8	Dis.-Seagrams	3,285	12	12	9	9	− 3
91	87	Dom. Tar p.	10	87½	...	...	...	− 1
113	91	Duf. Pav. pfd.	65	91	92	91	92	− 1
28	8	Durant Motors	455	9	9	8	8	− 1½
32	17	Eng. Elc. B. p.	195	24	25	24	25	unch
20	18	Ed.-C. Dairy c.	35	18	...	...	...	− 2
90	90	Do., pfd.	70	90	...	...	...	unch
95½	90	Firstbrook p.	50	90	...	...	...	− 3
13.5	100	Foothills Oil	200	100	160	100	160	− 1.15
377	150	Goodyear T. c.	280	150	170	150	160	− 30
89¾	31	Ham. Bridge	100	32	32	31	31	− 4
27.00	3.15	Home Oil	200	11.00	11.00	10.75	10.75	− 2.25
85½	64	Honey Dew p.	5	69	...	...	...	− 1
41	26	Imperial Oil	30,638	20½	31	26	30	− 2
30	18	Internat. Pete	43,370	18⅞	22	18	19	− 3
11½	9	Imp. Tob.	340	10	10	9¾	10	− ½
45	25	McColl-Fronc.c.	10	25	...	...	...	− 4
140½	39¾	Nat. Steel Car	100	39¾	...	...	...	− ¾
139	80½	Pow. Cor. c.	346	92	92	80½	83¼	− 12
25½	17	Prairie Oils	30	17	...	...	...	unch
...	...	Quebec	100	2.00	...	...	...	...
210	75	Royalite	15	75	...	...	...	unch

1929 High	Low	Stocks	Sales	Open	High	Low	Cl'se	Net Ch'ge
89	35	Serv. Stat. A.	3,455	53	54	35	45	– 10
111½	68¾	Shawinigan	105	76¼	79½	75¾	79	– 8
39	24½	Stan. Pav. & M. c.	465	28	28	24½	25	– 3
45½	22	Super, O.N.V. . . .	665	28	30	22	23	– 7¼
44	30	Do. com. V.T. . .	10	30	. . .	. . .	. . .	– ½
62	40	Tamblyn, com. . .	10	55	. . .	. . .	. . .	– 1
102	99	Do. pref.	10	99	. . .	. . .	. . .	unch
39	15	Waterloo Mfg. . .	1,010	17	17	15	16	– 2
		Mines						
66¼	18	Coast Copper . . .	50	18	. . .	. . .	. . .	– 7
70.00	26.50	Noranda	17,606	34.50	34.50	26.50	26.75	– 13.25
9.80	4.05	Sherritt-Gordon .	100	4.05	. . .	. . .	. . .	– 1.55
10.25	5.00	Teck-Hughes . . .	600	5.15	. . .	. . .	. . .	– 35

Total sales: 332,900 shares
(From the *Mail and Empire*, October 30, 1929.)

Quotations from the Standard Stock and Mining Exchange, Tuesday, October 29, 1929

1929 High	Low	Stocks	Sales	Open	High	Low	Cl'se	Net Ch'ge
25	4½	Aconda.	9,300	8	10	8	8	unch
3.65	26	Ajax Oil	69,400	1.42	1.42	1.31	1.36	– 9
5.25	1.65	Alta. Pac. Con. . .	19,310	2.05	2.08	1.65	1.80	– 30
48	13	Amity Copper . .	5,500	14	15	13	15	+ 1
3.75	1.00	Amulet	79,865	2.35	2.40	1.85	2.00	– 45
20	5	Area	4,000	8	8½	8	8	– ½
1.73	15	Arno	63,400	20	20	15	17	– 3
95	31	Acme	9,900	60	60	51	55	– 6½
3.65	2.00	Admiral	50	2.00	. . .	. . .	. . .	unch
4⅞	3¼	Baldwin	8,500	3½	3½	3¼	3¼	unch
44	16	Barry-Holl.	24,000	18	18	17	18	– 1½
6.50	2.75	Base Metals	12,445	4.40	4.40	2.75	3.50	– 1.00
38¾	3	Bathurst	2,600	5	5	4	5	unch
72	25	Bedford	2,600	30	30	25	25	– 12
60	9	Bidgood	9,500	15	15½	13	13	– 3
5.50	1.00	Calmont Oil	21,325	1.19	1.19	1.00	1.05	– 15
1.40	70	Canam Metals . . .	700	70	. . .	. . .	. . .	– 25
10	5	Capitol Silver . . .	1,500	5	. . .	. . .	. . .	unch
40	28	Castle-Treth. . . .	11,100	30	30	29½	29½	+ ½
48	6	Clericy	500	6	. . .	. . .	. . .	unch
1.92	49	Columario	10,050	1.82	1.82	49	49	– 1.35
1.53	50	Com. Pete	3,700	50	60	50	60	– 30
11.25	4.40	Dome Mines	20,176	7.00	7.00	4.40	6.25	– 2.15
8	2	Duprat	2,700	3½	3½	3¼	3¼	+ ¼
16.50	4.75	Falconbridge	8,265	6.75	6.75	4.75	6.15	– 1.60
83	62	Goldfield	8,600	75	75	62	62	– 13
50	1¼	Graham-Bous . . .	1,500	2	2	1¼	1¼	– ¾

1929 High	Low	Stocks	Sales	Open	High	Low	Cl'se	Net Ch'ge
49	14	Grand Rouyn . . .	20,005	18	18	14½	15	− 4
1.00	14½	Grandview	900	20	20	14½	14½	− 5½
1.40	65	Howey Gold	64,575	85	85	65	65	− 21
10.00	1.00	Hollinger Cons. .	9,330	5.40	5.40	4.00	4.60	− 80
62	30	Keeley	1,500	40	40	30	30	− 12
1.92	47	Kirkland Lake . . .	22,425	60	60	47	50	− 11
19	2	Kirkland Prem. . .	1,000	2½	. . .	. . .	. . .	unch
30	8½	Kootenay Flor. . .	8,100	9	10	8½	8½	− 1½
. . .	. . .	Lake Shore	15,551	20.00	20.00	13.00	16.75	− 3.35
15.75	1.50	Mayland Oil	2,560	2.35	2.35	1.50	2.00	− 50
1.14	3	Malartic Gold . . .	1,700	3	4	3	4	+ ½
76	11	Manitoba Basin . .	41,710	13	14	11	14	unch
1.25	50	Mercury	850	50	. . .	. . .	. . .	unch
70	30	McDougall	5,600	30	33	30	30	− 5
24.00	13.75	McIntyre	6,610	14.75	14.75	13.75	13.75	− 1.25
6.02	2.75	Mining Corp. . . .	24,200	3.50	3.50	2.75	2.80	− 70
30	2	Moffatt H., New .	1,500	3	3¼	3	3¼	+ ¼
67	3½	Murphy	1,000	4	. . .	. . .	. . .	+ ½
94	15	Newbec	125,180	20	22	15	18	− 5
6	6	Night Hawk	20,000	5½	. . .	. . .	. . .	unch
3.90	2.00	Nipissing	3,895	2.10	2.10	2.00	2.00	− 15
70.00	27.00	Noranda	85,000	37.50	37.75	27.00	27.00	− 11.25
. . .	. . .	Nor. Canada	1,000	30	. . .	. . .	. . .	unch
68	7	Old Colony	1,000	9	. . .	. . .	. . .	− 2
37	11½	Peterson Cob. . . .	2,300	17	. . .	. . .	. . .	− 3
68	17	Pioneer M. C. . . .	3,400	22	22	20	20	− 5
2.35	1.50	Premier Gold . . .	6,035	1.65	1.65	1.50	1.50	− 15
26½	10	San Antonio	11,300	11	13	10	13	unch
9.90	4.00	Sherritt-Gord. . .	118,993	5.00	5.00	4.00	4.05	− 1.10
1.60	48½	Siscoe	43,250	65	65	50	53	. . .
8.00	1.00	S.W. Pete	8,625	1.25	1.25	1.00	1.00	− 45
15	5	Stadacona	6,600	5	. . .	. . .	. . .	− ½
2.75	68	Sterling Pac.	5,125	85	85	68	68	− 32
93	10	St. Anthony	1,200	12	. . .	. . .	. . .	+ 2
13.75	3.75	Sudbury Basin . . .	64,100	6.00	6.00	3.75	4.25	− 1.30
. . .	. . .	Sylvanite	4,500	55	58	55	55	unch
10.25	4.75	Teck-Hughes . . .	68,025	5.35	5.40	4.75	5.00	− 25
50	6	Thom. Cadillac . .	500	6	. . .	. . .	. . .	unch
3.50	1.00	Towagmac	1,745	1.10	1.15	1.00	1.00	− 15
20	10	The Petrol Oil . .	500	13	. . .	. . .	. . .	− 2
18.50	7.25	Treadwell, c. . . .	150	7.25	. . .	. . .	. . .	− 50
1.26	55	Vipond. Con. . . .	24,200	62	62	58	60	− 7
70	12	Wainwell Oils . . .	40,100	14¼	14¼	12	13	− 1¼
8.30	1.50	Waite-Acker	1,100	3.50	3.50	3.40	3.40	− 60
2.95	1.25	Wright-Harg. . . .	26,410	1.45	1.45	1.25	1.25	− 25

UNLISTED

3.90	1.70	Abana	67,275	1.38	1.38	1.15	1.25	− 15
6.75	90	Assoc. Oil & G. .	12,527	1.35	1.35	90	1.10	− 25

1929

High	Low	Stocks	Sales	Open	High	Low	Cl'se	Net Ch'ge
4.75	45	Baltac	5,520	60	60	45	45	– 20
71.55	41.00	B.A. Oil	554	44.00	44.00	41.00	41.00	– 11
2.46	45	Big Missouri	87,100	70	73	45	55	– 18
8.50	4.05	Bwana M'Kub ...	12,800	6.25	6.25	5.75	5.75	– 85
11.25	1.75	Calgary & Ed. ...	8,054	2.10	2.10	1.75	1.75	– 85
80	20	Cen. Manitoba ..	6,200	24	24	20	20	– 6
21.50	7.25	Chem. Res.	1,830	8.25	8.25	7.25	7.25	– 1.00
66.25	20.00	Coast Copper ...	25	20.00	...	...	...	– 3.00
10.75	1.15	Dalhousie Oil ...	8,865	1.60	1.60	1.15	1.25	– 40
4.75	90	Eastcrest	13,100	1.25	1.25	90	90	– 35
9.50	1.60	Foothill	1,375	2.20	2.20	1.60	1.75	– 50
27.00	9.75	Home Oil	10,700	12.40	12.40	9.75	10.60	– 1.80
23.00	10.00	Hudson Bay	15,995	12.00	12.50	10.00	11.00	– 2.00
41.00	27.00	Imperial O., N. ..	1,885	30.50	30.50	27.00	28.75	– 3.75
29.75	19.00	Inter. Pete. N. ...	1,220	21.30	21.30	19.00	20.25	– 3.75
73.00	30.00	I. Nickel (Can.) .	51,134	36.00	38.25	30.00	30.00	– 9.00
36	1¼	Jackson Man. ...	1,000	2½	...	...	...	+ ½
1.80	25	Mandy Mines ...	3,300	30	30	25	25	– 9
1.05	19	Osisko	4,500	20	20	19	20	– 10
16.95	2.40	Pend Oreille	11,750	2.80	2.80	2.40	2.45	– 35
200.00	75.00	Royalite	10	75.00	...	...	...	– 13
14.85	3.50	Ventures	7,740	4.50	4.50	3.50	3.75	– 75

Sales: 1,743,592
(From the *Mail and Empire*, October 30, 1929.)

Quotations from the Montreal Stock Exchange, Tuesday, October 29, 1929

Morning Transactions

Abitibi—205 at 40, 35 at 40½, 40 at 41, 25 at 40½, 50 at 40¾, 60 at 40, 20 at 41, 100 at 44½.

Alberta Grain, class "A"—10 at 35, 50 at 34.

Asbestos—85 at 4½, 50 at 4¼.

Atlantic Sugar—90 at 8.

Brazilian—10,000 at 50, 100 at 49¾, 125 at 49½, 50 at 49½, 2,000 at 49, 200 at 48¾, 225 at 48½, 50 at 48¼, 505 at 48, 2,737 at 47½, 55 at 47¼, 680 at 47, 10 at 46¼, 3,760 at 46, 510 at 45¼, 1,140 at 45, 100 at 44¾, 70 at 44¼, 5,860 at 44, 100 at 43¾, 1,000 at 43½, 585 at 43¼, 2,731 at 43, 165 at 42¾, 50 at 42½, 2,135 at 42, 500 at 41¾, 260 at 41½, 2,020 at 41, 25 at 40¾, 2,350 at 40½, 4,110 at 40, 20 at 39 ⅞, 3,675 at 39½, 5,185 at 39, 2,230 at 40, 575 at 40½, 145 at 41, 125 at 41½, 100 at 41¾, 65 at 42, 15 at 42½, 3,950 at 43, 1,590 at 43¼, 260 at 43½, 24 at 43¾, 3,300 at 44, 175 at 44¼, 100 at 44½, 120 at 45, 30 at 45½, 690 at 45¾, 25 at 45⅞, 2,200 at 46, 350 at 46½, 385 at 46¾, 4,190 at 47,675 at 47¼, 100 at 47½, 75 at 46,250 at 45¾, 57 at 45, 25 at 44¾, 255 at 44½, 210 at 44¼, 1,160 at 44, 710 at 43¾, 100 at 43½, 1,800 at 43,500 at 42¾, 1,815 at 42½, 50 at 42½, 5,453 at 42,1,000 at 41½,1,900 at 41¼, 2,225 at 41, 5 at 40⅝, 3,680 at 40½, 10 at 40¼, 50 at 40 ⅛, 72 at 40.

Bell Telephone—20 at 159, 50 at 158, 5 at 157½, 10 at 158, 7 at 157, 8 at 159.

Bell Telephone Rights—10 at 5.00, 56 at 4.50, 13 at 4.00.

B.C. Packers—165 at 10.

British Columbia Power, Class "A"—10 at 40, 55 at 40½, 40 at 41, 75 at 40½, 50 at 41½, 105 at 41, 50 at 42, 265 at 41, 100 at 40½, 955 at 41.

British Columbia Power, Class "B"—150 at 24, 145 at 22, 25 at 25.

Brompton—15 at 34, 75 at 33, 10 at 34, 125 at 33, 50 at 32½, 75 at 33, 25 at 34, 20 at 32¾, 35 at 33.

Bruck Silk—50 at 25, 50 at 24½, 25 at 25, 25 at 24½, 100 at 25, 150 at 24½, 45 at 25, 10 at 24, 35 at 25.

Building Prod.—25 at 28.

Can. Alcohol—760 at 10, 10 at 10¼, 75 at 10, 50 at 10¼, 225 at 10, 130 at 10¼, 1,200 at 10, 20 at 10½, 100 at 10, 90 at 10¼, 10 at 10½, 30 at 10.

Can. Brewing—140 at 8, 15 at 8¼, 295 at 8, 10 at 8¼.

Can. Bronze—10 at 52, 25 at 53.

Can. Car & Foundry (New)—100 at 23½, 5 at 20½, 405 at 20, 20 at 21, 210 at 20, 380 at 21, 100 at 20, 30 at 21, 50 at 20, 25 at 20¼, 75 at 19, 845 at 20, 125 at 19, 50 at 20, 160 at 21, 435 at 20.

Can. Cement—5 at 20, 400 at 21, 25 at 19, 20 at 20¼, 5 at 20¾.

Can. Forgings, Class "A"—25 at 16.

Can. Gypsum & A—120 at 24, 100 at 23, 175 at 24, 50 at 23.

Can. Power & Paper—1,555 at 26, 50 at 25⅛, 75 at 25½, 326 at 26, 10 at 25, 215 at 24, 50 at 25, 35 at 24, 35 at 25, 75 at 24, 25 at 25, 400 at 24, 20 at 23½, 10 at 23¾,25 at 24⅜, 205 at 24, 100 at 25, 25 at 25, 215 at 26, 26 at 24½, 15 at 24.

Can. Steamships—75 at 20.

Can. Wire & Cable, Class "B"—35 at 32.

Cockshutt Plow—110 at 24, 5 at 23½, 30 at 24, 10 at 26, 20 at 24, 174 at 22, 60 at 21, 25 at 20, 25 at 21, 20 at 19, 55 at 20, 55 at 21.

Con. Smelters—110 at 295, 19 at 280, 30 at 275, 35 at 265, 30 at 270, 95 at 265, 25 at 260, 575 at 250, 40 at 240, 40 at 250, 10 at 260.

Dom. Bridge—1,480 at 80, 225 at 78, 25 at 77, 40 at 76½, 200 at 75, 25 at 74, 170 at 73, 125 at 72, 10 at 71, 195 at 70, 440 at 69, 400 at 70, 50 at 71, 50 at 70†, 60 at 69, 90 at 70, 100 at 68, 25 at 70, 30 at 75, 25 at 70, 50 at 69, 155 at 68½, 41 at 68, 80 at 68½, 100 at 69, 125 at 69¼, 110 at 69, 10 at 66, 10 at 67, 60 at 70, 270 at 69, 170 at 70, 285 at 69, 15 at 68½, 10 at 68, 10 at 70.

Dom. Glass—40 at 85, 60 at 86, 200 at 80, 170 at 85.

Donnacona—70 at 24.

East Kootenay—1 at 25.

Famous Players—20 at 45, 75 at 43, 5 at 40, 225 at 45, 75 at 41, 105 at 40, 485 at 41, 30 at 43, 25 at 44½, 25 at 38, 5 at 39, 15 at 39½, 5 at 40.

Fraser—50 at 33, 20 at 34, 1 at 36, 50 at 30.

Gen. Steel Wares—290 at 25, 25 at 22, 40 at 25, 25 at 23, 145 at 22, 25 at 21, 410 at 20, 190 at 22, 50 at 23, 5 at 21.

Gurd—25 at 30†, 10 at 28.

Hamilton Bridge—120 at 35, 75 at 34, 125 at 30, 25 at 33.

Int. Nickel of C.—7, 312 at 35, 1,505 at 34½, 5,450 at 34, 10 at 33½, 10 at 33¼, 3,076 at 33, 140 at 32¾ 1,075 at 32½, 5,400 at 32, 75 at 31⅞, 90 at 31¾, 280 at 31½, 560 at 31, 50 at 30¾, 220 at 30½, 8,886 at 30, 50 at 29⅞, 500 at 29½, 5,105 at 30, 350 at 30½, 1,810 at 31, 25 at 31¼, 375 at 31½, 880 at 31¾, 4,356 at 32, 755 at 32¼, 585 at 32½, 700 at 32⅝, 7,710 at 33, 425 at 33¼, 890 at 33½, 30 at 33¾, 65 at 34, 50 at 34½, 900 at 33½, 200 at 33¼, 11,375 at 33, 305 at 32¾, 3,105 at 32½, 150 at 32¼, 1,455 at 32, 25 at 31⅞, 15 at 31¾, 60 at 31½, 1,300 at 31, 550 at 33½, 6,895 at 33, 10 at 32⅞, 10 at 32¾, 780 at 32½, 1,400 at 32¼, 12,400 at 32, 35 at 31⅞, 1,615 at 31¾, 1,120 at 31½, 10 at 31¼, 200 at 31, 360 at 30.

Int. Power—15 at 19.

Lake of Woods—35 at 47, 15 at 40, 10 at 50, 132 at 48.

Lindsay, C.W.—125 at 26.

Massey-Harris—30 at 39, 5 at 40, 65 at 39, 195 at 39¼, 595 at 39, 295 at 38, 25 at 38½, 210 at 38, 5 at 34, 5 at 34½, 30 at 35, 450 at 39, 55 at 39¼, 25 at 38, 190 at 39, 20 at 36, 5 at 38, 10 at 39, 10 at 38.

McColl-Frontenac—1,575 at 27, 450 at 26½, 495 at 26, 1,000 at 25, 50 at 26, 610 at 25, 290 at 26, 165 at 25, 255 at 26, 25 at 25½, 275 at 25.

Mont. Power—560 at 143, 385 at 141, 425 at 140, 75 at 143, 25 at 139, 15 at 137½, 55 at 137, 15 at 138, 107 at 139, 130 at 140, 170 at 139, 35 at 136, 85 at 135, 10 at 135½, 370 at 138, 95 at 137, 60 at 137½, 65 at 138, 25 at 139, 15 at 140, 235 at 138, 385 at 137, 100 at 136, 400 at 137⅛, 50 at 137, 100 at 136, 95 at 135, 205 at 138, 50 at 140, 50 at 139, 375 at 138, 140 at 137½, 320 at 137, 75 at 136, 115 at 135, 50 at 136, 50 at 137, 100 at 137⅛, 20 at 135, 20 at 134½, 10 at 136, 15 at 134, 10 at

132, 20 at 133, 330 at 135, 25 at 134½, 10 at 134¼, 100 at 126, 10 at 124, 50 at 126, 25 at 129, 25 at 130, 50 at 135, 5 at 138, 10 at 143, 30 at 135, 15 at 134, 32 at 133, 295 at 130, 35 at 129, 90 at 128, 40 at 127, 60 at 126, 90 at 125, 3 at 124.

Nat. Breweries—285 at 120, 80 at 118, 85 at 120.

Nat. Steel Car—25 at 50.

Niagara Wire—25 at 20.

Power Corp.—25 at 92, 11½ at 93, 75 at 90, 305 at 93, 35 at 89, 150 at 90, 475 at 88, 155 at 90, 35 at 89, 275 at 88, 10 at 88½, 20 at 87½, 200 at 89, 500 at 90, 110 at 88, 30 at 87, 25 at 85, 50 at 86½, 101 at 86, 180 at 85½, 25 at 87, 10 at 85, 25 at 84, 15 at 82, 50 at 86½, 55 at 87, 65 at 87½, 100 at 82½, 200 at 81½, 5 at 81, 70 at 88, 225 at 82, 25 at 87, 25 at 81, 15 at 81½, 225 at 90, 25 at 89, 870 at 88, 5 at 87, 15 at 84, 5 at 87, 105-100 at 90.

Shawinigan—297 at 81, 75 at 80, 110 at 80½, 100 at 80¼, 235 at 80½, 95 at 79, 100 at 80¼, 200 at 80, 75 at 79¼, 110 at 80½, 125 at 80, 45 at 76, 10 at 75, 25 at 77, 5 at 88, 530 at 80, 30 at 78½, 50 at 77¼, 456 at 77, 330 at 76, 100 at 79½, 30 at 80, 31 at 75, 120 at 76½, 16 at 76, 385 at 77, 294 at 76, 100 at 77¼, 50 at 78, 50 at 77½, 275 at 76, 50 at 78, 650 at 80, 10 at 78½, 100 at 78, 170 at 77½, 515 at 77, 50 at 76½, 50 at 76, 130 at 75¼, 25 at 75, 31 at 76, 126 at 77, 26 at 78, 20 at 76¼, 350 at 76, 460 at 77, 5 at 73½, 225 at 77, 50 at 74, 280 at 77, 25 at 76¼, 35 at 76, 20 at 75, 10 at 77, 60 at 75, 12 at 77, 15 at 76, 15 at 77, 20 at 78, 13 at 77, 10 at 76, 15 at 77½, 10 at 78, 15 at 77¼, 10 at 77.

Price—180 at 90, 505 at 88.

Quebec Power—25 at 72, 10 at 73, 20 at 70, 20 at 72, 55 at 70, 350 at 69, 25 at 67, 25 at 70, 15 at 68, 25 at 70, 40 at 67.

Sher. Williams—135 at 40.

S. Can. Power—70 at 42, 50 at 43, 30 at 42.

Steel of Canada—445 at 50, 25 at 49, 40 at 48, 50 at 48½, 130 at 49, 10 at 48, 10 at 49, 45 at 48, 125 at 49, 25 at 47, 100 at 45, 100 at 48, 50 at 47, 100 at 46, 85 at 47, 25 at 48, 90 at 48¼, 25 at 48, 100 at 49, 15 at 48¼, 50 at 48½, 50 at 50, 10 at 45, 20 at 48¼, 15 at 48.

St. Law. Paper—200 at 15.

Vise Biscuit—10 at 16¼.

Winnipeg—50 at 56, 40 at 60, 15 at 50, 10 at 51¼, 20 at 50, 45 at 52, . . . at . . ., 50 at 56, 25 at 55, 10 at 56, 10 at 56, 10 at 54, 10 at 52.

PREFERRED

Abitibi—530 at 60.

Asbestos—45 at 17.

Brit. Empire Ind.—20 at 5½.

Can. Car & Fdr. (New)—100 at 24, 150 at 25¼, 90 at 24½, 945 at 25, 795 at 25, 86 at 24, 175 at 25, 46 at 24, 415 at 25, 165 at 24½, 40 at 25.

Can. Cement—25 at 95, 25 at 94½, 25 at 95½.

Can. Steamships—40 at 75, 10 at 77, 41 at 75.

Dom. Steel Corp.—5 at 49½, 10 at 41.

Ham. Bridge—55 at 89.

Sher. Williams—25 at 118½.

Steel of Canada—25 at 43.

BANKS

Canadienne—9 at 171¼, 25 at 171.

Montreal—57 at 330, 28 at 328.

Nova Scotia—25 at 388.

Royal—29 at 329, 30 at 326, 10 at 329.

BONDS

C. Pow. & Paper Debentures—4,000 at 78¼.

McNish & Co. Debentures—$200 at 3.75.

Afternoon Transactions

Abitibi P. & P.—20 at 41, 150 at 40¾, 20 at 42, 25 at 40, 35 at 40½, 75 at 40, 25 at 40½, 60 at 41, 10 at 40½, 35 at 41, 25 at 40¾, 360 at 40, 25 at 40¼, 40 at 40½, 60 at 40, 100 at 41, 75 at 40, 75 at 40½, 100 at 41.

Alberta Grain Class "A"—40 at 34, 75 at 33, 100 at 31, 150 at 33, 50 at 35, 35 at 36, 35 at 31, 325 at 30, 30 at 30½, 285 at 30, 100 at 33¼, 75 at 33, 5 at 34, 25 at 31.

Asbestos Corp.—105 at 4¼, 235 at 4, 100 at 3½.

Bell Telephone—4 at 154, 25 at 157, 5 at 152, 119 at 150, 29 at 153, 30 at 151, 20 at 156, 29 at 154, 55 at 156, 10 at 151.

Bell Tel. Rights—35 at 4.00, 11 at 4.25, 1,890 at 4.50, 295 at 4.25, 3 at 4.50, 510 at 4.00.

Brazilian—15 at 42½, 10 at 42¼, 741 at 42, 775 at 41¾, 500 at 41½, 200 at 41⅛, 3,800 at 41, 625 at 40½, 375 at 40¼, 810 at 40⅛, 1,746 at 40, 2,208 at 41, 825 at 41⅛, 405 at 41¼, 100 at 41⅜, 1,881 at 41½, 250 at 41¾, 60 at 41½, 10,032 at 42, 225 at 42⅛, 410 at 42¼, 60 at 43, 1,450 at 42¼, 1,395 at 42½, 270 at 42⅜,

1,055 at 42⅞, 2,730 at 43, 100 at 43⅛, 260 at 43¼, 1,331 at 43½, 450 at 43¾, 895 at 44, 90 at 44¼, 485 at 44½, 535 at 44¾, 1,377 at 45, 50 at 45¼, 340 at 45½, 1,126 at 45½, 375 at 43¾, 25 at 45⅞, 170 at 48, 1,409 at 42¾, 1,786 at 43, 65 at 43⅛, 180 at 43¼, 25 at 43¾, 140 at 43½, 50 at 43⅜, 1,290 at 43¾, 40 at 44, 25 at 44⅜, 520 at 41½, 35 at 41⅝, 6,190 at 41, 150 at 41⅛, 625 at 41¼, 1,380 at 41½, 250 at 41¾, 125 at 41⅞, 3,730 at 42, 25 at 42⅛, 1,950 at 42¼, 750 at 42½, 2,055 at 42¾, 765 at 43, 100 at 43¼, 455 at 43½.

B.C. Packers—450 at 10.

B.C. Power "A"—150 at 41, 10 at 40, 760 at 41, 100 at 40½, 110 at 41, 15 at 40½, 30 at 41¾, 425 at 41, 15 at 40, 10 at 40½, 110 at 40¼, 75 at 41, 15 at 40½, 80 at 40¼, 100 at 40, 25 at 39½, 125 at 39, 25 at 40.

B.C. Power "B"—156 at 23, 175 at 25, 35 at 23¼, 25 at 23, 50 at 23¼.

Brompton—175 at 32¼, 10 at 32, 50 at 33, 70 at 32, 25 at 31½, 10 at 28, 50 at 29, 200 at 27½, 25 at 29, 25 at 28, 25 at 28½, 25 at 27½, 40 at 26¾, 20 at 27, 75 at 26¾.

Bruck Silk—35 at 24, 50 at 23, 100 at 23½, 450 at 22½, 300 at 22.

Building Prod.—25 at 28, 25 at 27½.

Can. Alcohol—150 at 10, 30 at 10½, 1,110 at 10, 305 at 9½, 20 at 9, 25 at 9½, 515 at 10, 50 at 10¼, 72 at 10, 165 at 11, 155 at 10½.

C. Brew Corp.—40 at 6, 10 at 8, 85 at 6, 75 at 8, 80 at 6, 95 at 8.

Can. Bronze—40 at 50, 65 at 47, 25 at 43, 85 at 44, 25 at 45, 105 at 46, 140 at 49, 105 at 47, 425 at 40, 100 at 40¼, 100 at 40, 25 at 43, 25 at 40, 25 at 42.

Can. Car New—340 at 20, 20 at 19, 25 at 20½, 1,175 at 20, 65 at 19¾, 200 at 19¼, 910 at 19, 760 at 19½, 265 at 20, 176 at 19½, 380 at 19, 95 at 21, 50 at 20½, 200 at 20, 65 at 21, 60 at 20½, 660 at 20.

Can. Car & Fdy.—60 at 78.

Can. Cement—10 at 17, 60 at 14, 10 at 15, 30 at 14½, 100 at 14, 25 at 14½, 240 at 14, 10 at 14¼, 250 at 14, 15 at 14¼, 295 at 14.

C. Power & Paper—100 at 25, 205 at 24, 25 at 23½, 10 at 23, 45 at 24, 25 at 23¾, 200 at 23½, 25 at 23⅛, 1,090 at 23, 50 at 22, 331 at 21, 100 at 20, 50 at 21, 10 at 21⅛, 10 at 20¼, 225 at 21½, 535 at 22, 620 at 21, 135 at 22, 5 at 23, 40 at 21¼, 210 at 21½, 270 at 22, 25 at 22⅛, 125 at 22¼, 25 at 22, 295 at 22½, 25 at 22¼, 175 at 22.

C. Forgings "A"—50 at 16.

C. Gypsum & A—65 at 20, 15 at 19, 70 at 20, 100 at 22, 35 at 19, 125 at 18½, 1,505 at 18, 10 at 19.

C. Steamships—600 at 20.

Cockshutt Plow—35 at 20, 10 at 18, 185 at 19, 670 at 18, 25 at 17⅞, 45 at 17½, 15 at 15, 75 at 18, 310 at 17, 290 at 17½, 10 at 17¼, 35 at 16, 105 at 16½, 25 at 17, 360 at 16½, 110 at 17, 40 at 17½, 40 at 18, 50 at 18¼, 310 at 18, 25 at 19, 175 at 18.

Cons. Smelters—81 at 250, 5 at 240, 25 at 250, 25 at 240, 250 at 250, 60 at 235, 130 at 230, 11 at 235, 70 at 240, 235 at 235, 5 at 230, 200 at 235, 15 at 240, 15 at 235.

Dom. Bridge—1,060 at 70, 130 at 69, 25 at 68⅞, 670 at 68, 85 at 67, 100 at 66, 195 at 65½, 750 at 65, 100 at 64¾. 25 at 64½, 215 at 64, 50 at 63½, 630 at 64, 45 at 65, 35 at 67, 730 at 68, 220 at 69, 17 at 65, 50 at 64½, 565 at 64, 40 at 63½, 650 at 63, 382 at 68, 135 at 68¼, 105 at 68½, 760 at 68, 135 at 67½, 40 at 67, 25 at 66, 50 at 65½, 225 at 65.

Dom. Textile—100 at 85, 50 at 80½, 120 at 84, 170 at 85, 20 at 84, 25 at 80, 10 at 83, 15 at 80.

F. Players—35 at 39½, 50 at 40, 10 at 38½, 80 at 38, 85 at 41, 15 at 40, 25 at 39½, 50 at 39, 25 at 38¼, 1,245 at 38, 75 at 37, 25 at 40, 25 at 41, 10 at 42, 120 at 41, 320 at 39, 10 at 40½, 75 at 40, 25 at 40½, 60 at 41, 60 at 40, 110 at 41, 15 at 40¾, 100 at 41, 175 at 40, 15 at 39, 25 at 40.

Donnacona P.—15 at 23, 15 at 24, 90 at 23, 35 at 24, 195 at 23.

Enmael & Heat—5 at 28.

Foundation Co.—25 at 18.

Fraser—15 at 28, 85 at 30.

Gurd—25 at 28½, 25 at 30.

G. Steel Wares—35 at 1, 65 at 20, 45 at 20½, 35 at 20⅛, 160 at 20, 50 at 19, 70 at 20, 5 at 21.

Int. Nickel of C.—1,025 at 33, 8,602 at 32, 185 at 31⅞, 1,785 at 31¾, 25 at 31⅝, 7,175 at 31½, 180 at 31¼, 1,615 at 31, 25 at 30¾, 1,565 at 30½, 660 at 30¼, 20 at 30, 2,000 at 30¼, 125 at 30½, 50 at 30¾, 100 at 30⅞, 1,125 at 31, 3,025 at 31⅛, 1,935 at 31¼, 3,595 at 31½, 180 at 31⅝, 2,345 at 31¾, 135 at 31⅞, 11,397 at 32, 1,280 at 32½, 770 at 32¾, 90 at 32⅞, 3,908 at 33, 75 at 33½, 775 at 33¼, 100 at 33¾, 2,135 at 33½, 380 at 33¼, 2,925 at 33, 510 at 32⅞, 1,450 at 32¾, 2,926 at 32½, 175 at 32⅞, 880 at

32¼, 2,860 at 32, 20 at 31⅞, 45 at 31¾, 45 at 31¾, 210 at 31½, 535 at 31¼, 4,550 at 31, 1,485 at 30⅞, 105 at 30⅝, 80 at 30¾, 3,365 at 30¼, 2,955 at 30⅛, 15,100 at 30, 3,500 at 30½, 1,065 at 30¾.

Hamilton Bridge—50 at 30, 5 at 30¼, 25 at 28, 80 at 30, 125 at 28, 10 at 27, 50 at 27½, 100 at 25, 15 at 26, 200 at 25.

Hollinger—100 at 4.50.

Int. Power—25 at 19, 200 at 20, 50 at 18, 46 at 19, 10 at 18.

Lake of Woods—10 at 45, 15 at 47, 25 at 46, 10 at 47, 120 at 45, 5 at 46, 100 at 45.

Massey-Harris—25 at 38, 20 at 35, 30 at 34, 10 at 33, 25 at 37, 200 at 36, 300 at 35, 1,440 at 34, 515 at 33, 40 at 32½, 2,120 at 33, 295 at 33¼, 35 at 33¼, 430 at 34, 50 at 36, 75 at 33½, 175 at 35, 20 at 36, 55 at 36¼, 760 at 36, 65 at 35½, 85 at 35, 150 at 35½.

McColl-Frontenac—380 at 25, 10 at 24¼, 795 at 23, 480 at 25, 20 at 24½, 635 at 24¼, 540 at 24, 113 at 23½, 240 at 23, 80 at 23½, 10 at 23¼, 25 at 23½, 25 at 23¼, 25 at 24, 5 at 23, 15 at 23⅛, 110 at 23¼, 85 at 24, 50 at 23½, 2,160 at 23, 1,000 at 22.

Mitchell, J.S.—50 at 35.

Mont. Telegraph—50 at 48.

Mont. Power—25 at 133, 25 at 131, 145 at 129, 45 at 128, 20 at 127, 930 at 126, 922 at 125, 115 at 124½, 462 at 124, 1 at 123, 390 at 122, 210 at 121, 5 at 120½, 10 at 120¼, 475 at 120, 35 at 125, 30 at 128, 440 at 130, 105 at 131, 50 at 132, 151 at 133, 145 at 134, 60 at 135, 50 at 136, 100 at 137, 35 at 138, 15 at 135, 35 at 127, 90 at 126, 145 at 125, 235 at 124, 10 at 123, 20 at 122, 20 at 121, 60 at 120, 20 at 125, 310 at 130, 33 at 131, 20 at 131½, 150 at 132, 85 at 133, 75 at 133¾, 95 at 134, 30 at 135, 130 at 130, 105 at 129, 30 at 128, 75 at 127, 10 at 126, 50 at 128, 265 at 125.

Nat. Breweries—800 at 118, 100 at 117, 500 at 116,500 at 113, 150 at 114, 50 at 111, 395 at 110, 75 at 113, 895 at 119, 150 at 111, 25 at 110¾, 85 at 110, 140 at 111, 160 at 113.

Nat. Steel Car—15 at 46, 885 at 40, 163 at 45, 190 at 44, 25 at 41, 795 at 40.

Ogilvie Milling—15 at 550, 10 at 500.

Port Alfred—225 at 60.

Power Corp.—50 at 84, 150 at 83, 175 at 82, 51 at 81, 35 at 80, 25 at 85, 85 at 88, 50 at 87½, 160 at 83½, 85 at 82, 100 at 81½, 300 at 81, 150 at 80½, 100 at 80¼, 2,220 at 80, 15 at 79, 106 at 81, 170 at 80, 35 at 82, 100 at 83, 125 at 84, 50 at 85, 10 at 85½, 25 at 86, 15 at 87, 50 at 87½, 50 at 80½, 100 at 80, 355 at 79, 25 at 82, 10 at 85, 100 at 87½, 20 at 87, 250 at 82, 402 at 85, 50 at 86, 50 at 83, 20 at 82, 135 at 81, 130 at 80, 100 at 85.

Price Bros.—20 at 86, 25 at 88, 150 at 83, 135 at 84.

Quebec Power—10 at 65, 30 at 65½, 105 at 65, 10 at 63, 80 at 60, 150 at 63, 90 at 63, 225 at 63, 10 at 63½, 125 at 63, 225 at 62, 60 at 62, 70 at 64, 150 at 64, 80 at 65, 65 at 65, 145 at 63, 63 at 62, 35 at 65.

Que. Pow. Rights—5 at 200, 165 at 1.50.

Shawinigan—75 at 78, 235 at 77, 10 at 75, 15 at 74, 10 at 73¾, 25 at 73, 35 at 72, 25 at 77, 375 at 76, 1,805 at 75, 355 at 74, 225 at 73¾, 125 at 73½, 160 at 73, 2,587 at 72, 200 at 71½, 400 at 71, 146 at 75, 150 at 77, 15 at 77½, 665 at 78, 90 at 78¼, 5 at 78½, 107 at 79, 200 at 80, 15 at 75, 155 at 73, 55 at 72½, 912 at 72, 200 at 71½, 425 at 71, 45 at 75, 350 at 78, 124 at 78½, 85 at 79, 115 at 78½, 305 at 78, 10 at 78¼, 65 at 77½, 10 at 77, 188 at 76, 105 at 75, 125 at 74⅞, 10 at 74½, 150 at 74.

Sher. Williams—55 at 40.

Simon H. Sons—

South C. Power—20 at 40, 270 at 41, 120 at 40.

Steel of Canada—150 at 41, 525 at 40, 50 at 38, 1,896 at 35, 1,045 at 34, 200 at 36½, 285 at 37, 660 at 38, 100 at 38½, 50 at 38¾, 1,005 at 39, 50 at 39½. 190 at 40, 20 at 37, 90 at 36, 500 at 35, 640 at 39, 10 at 40, 50 at 39, 25 at 35, 175 at 39, 75 at 38, 20 at 37.

St. Law. Paper—30 at 15, 85 at 12.

Tooke Bros.—25 at 34.

Wayagamack—100 at 67, 100 at 62, 30 at 60, 15 at 62, 160 at 60, 10 at 62, 320 at 60.

Winnipeg—25 at 50, 40 at 47, 20 at 51, 150 at 50, 201 at 49, 300 at 48, 630 at 47, 10 at 48, 10 at 50, 50 at 47, 126 at 50, 20 at 51, 5 at 50½, 50 at 48, 115 at 47, 25 at 47½, 365 at 47, 40 at 51, 125 at 50, 20 at 50¼, 70 at 50, 60 at 51, 25 at 50½, 40 at 52, 70 at 51, 50 at 53, 10 at 57.

PREFERRED

Abitibi P. + P. 6%—220 at 80.

Belgo C. Paper—10 at 103.

B.E. Steel 2nd—105 at 5, 100 at 5½, 150 at 5, 25 at 4¾, 25 at 5.

C. Car and Foundry New—200 at 24, 100 at 23, 100 at 23½, 25 at 24, 115 at 23, 210 at 24, 235 at 23, 150 at 24, 25 at 23⅜, 25 at 25, 85 at 24, 100 at 23, 100 at 23½, 10 at 24, 150 at 23½, 245 at 23, 50 at 20, 130 at 23, 30 at 23½, 345 at 23, 25 at 24, 670 at 23½, 175 at 23½, 130 at 23.

C. Car & Foundry—25 at 75.

Can. Cement—25 at 94, 10 at 95½, 50 at 95, 10 at 93½, 5 at 95, 10 at 93½, 45 at 95.

C. Steamships—64 at 75, 50 at 75¼, 76 at 75, 25 at 75½, 20 at 75, 45 at 75.

Dom. Steel Corp.—15 at 40.

Hamilton Bridge—5 at 89.

Howard Smith—25 at 84, 10 at 85.

Int. Power—5 at 88.

Jamaica P. Ser.—100 at 112.

Nat. Breweries—500 at 127, 30 at 129, 200 at 130, 25 at 125.

Price Bros.—100 at 104.

Steel of Can.—520 at 40.

St. Maur. V. Corp—25 at 94.

BANKS

Commerce—171 at 280.

Montreal—8 at 328, 2 at 327½, 12 at 328, 3 at 329.

Nova Scotia—10 at 388.

Royal—43 at 322, 29 at 320, 176 at 320.

BONDS

Asbestos Corp. Gen. Mortgage—1,000 at 55.

C. Power and Paper debentures—3,500 at 78, 1,000 at 78½, 10,000 at 77, 3,000 at 76, 7,000 at 76½.

REFUNDING

1943—Tax, 2000 at 90.30.

Victory

1933—1000 at 100.66, 300 at 100.00, 20000 at 100.28.

1934—Tax—1000 at 100.25, 100 at 100.00, 100 at 100.00, 29000 at 100.20.

1937—1000 at 103.80.

(From the *Gazette*, October 30, 1929.)

Quotations from the Montreal Curb Market, Tuesday, October 29, 1929

Morning Transactions

Associated Oil—10 at 1.40, 400 at 1.00, 10 at 1.40.

British American Oil—5 at 49, 105 at 48, 20 at 47½, 25 at 46⅞, 25 at 43, 25 at 42, 290 at 41, 485 at 40, 90 at 39½, 50 at 39, 525 at 40, 105 at 41, 25 at 41½, 100 at 41, 125 at 40¾, 150 at 40½, 50 at 40½, 235 at 40, 50 at 41.

Can. Vinegars—25 at 32½.

Canadian Wineries—100 at 5.

Cosgrave Brewery—25 at 1.00.

Distillers-Seagrams—110 at 11½, 385 at 11, 90 at 10½, 83 at 10, 25 at 10¼, 10 at 10½, 20 at 11, 130 at 10, 155 at 10½, 70 at 10¼, 200 at 10.

Dryden Paper—160 at 19, 50 at 18½, 200 at 18, 160 at 17, 320 at 17¼, 135 at 17, 35 at 16¾, 10 at 17, 70 at 18.

Federal Distilleries—300 at 25.

Foreign Securities—150 at 32.

Home Oil—1900 at 12.25, 2010 at 12.00, 25 at 11.75, 100 at 11.80, 65 at 11.50, 35 at 11.00, 285 at 12.00, 5 at 11.75.

Hydro Electric—200 at 47.

Imperial Oil—660 at 31, 115 at 30½, 2790 at 30, 145 at 29⅞, 25 at 29¾, 355 at 29½, 397 at 29, 2035 at 28, 25 at 27¾, 720 at 27½, 170 at 27¼, 525 at 27, 50 at 26⅞, 40 at 26⅝, 30 at 26¾, 100 at 26½, 625 at 26, 210 at 25½, 1230 at 25, 225 at 24½, 125 at 25¼, 5250 at 26, 60 at 26¼, 75 at 26½, 10 at 26¾, 740 at 27, 50 at 27¼, 45 at 28*, 275 at 28¼, 175 at 28½, 10 at 28¾, 10 at 29, 100 at 28½, 250 at 28¼, 10 at 28, 10 at 27¾, 10 at 27, 40 at 25, 50 at 25½, 225 at 25¾, 1635 at 26, 55 at 26½, 50 at 26¾, 311 at 27.

Imperial Tobacco—950 at 10, 200 at 9¾, 525 at 10, 100 at 9⅝, 200 at 9⅛, 100 at 9¾.

International Paints—25 at 17.

Int. Petroleum—2180 at 20, 10 at 19⅞, 200 at 19, 545 at 18½, 175 at 18¼, 2885 at 18, 100 at 17¾, 425 at 17½, 460 at 17¼, 150 at 17, 60 at 18½, 10 at 18¾, 341 at 19, 25 at 19¼, 140 at

19½, 535 at 20, 17 at 20¼, 50 at 20½, 210 at 21, 10 at 20½, 100 at 19¾, 40 at 19¼, 225 at 19, 10 at 19½, 50 at 20, 575 at 21, 80 at 21½.

Int. Util. Class A—10 at 36, 55 at 35, 30 at 36.

National Distilleries—75 at 4.

Page-Hersey—25 at 98.

Sarnia Bridge, Class B—15 at 14.

Walker—25 at 9⅞, 375 at 10, 100 at 9¼, 375 at 9, 50 at 8¼, 60 at 8, 265 at 7, 50 at 6, 375 at 9½, 450 at 9¼, 450 at 9, 140 at 8½, 10 at 8.

Western Steel Products—5 at 40, 25 at 38, 25 at 36, 50 at 35.

PREFERRED

Dom. Tar and Chemical—25 at 87½, 25 at 87.

S. Can. Power—6 at 105½.

MINES

Noranda—50 at 36.99, 100 at 36.00, 100 at 35.35, 25 at 34.50, 320 at 33.00, 200 at 32.00, 205 at 31.00, 70 at 30.00, 15 at 30.75, 5 at 38.00, 100 at 34.00, 25 at 33.00, 100 at 31.00, 20 at 30.50, 650 at 30.00, 50 at 29.00, 175 at 29.00, 150 at 28.50, 772 at 28.00, 300 at 27.75, 770 at 27.50, 85 at 27.25, 645 at 27.00, 100 at 25.50, 80 at 26.00, 125 at 25.50, 100 at 25.25, 1950 at 25.00, 10 at 24.50, 75 at 25.25, 220 at 25.50, 600 at 26.00, 25 at 26.50, 140 at 27.00, 20 at 27.00, 5 at 28.00, 15 at 28.25, 40 at 28.50, 210 at 29.00, 100 at 29.75, 130 at 30.00, 85 at 29.50, 10 at 29.25, 100 at 29.00, 340 at 28.00, 20 at 27.00, 125 at 26.50, 75 at 27.50, 100 at 28.25, 850 at 28.50, 330 at 29.00, 50 at 29.50, 200 at 28.75, 945 at 28.50, 95 at 28.00, 25 at 28.25, 170 at 30.00, 10 at 27.50, 1995 at 27.00.

Abana—100 at 1.40, 5 at 1.50, 300 at 1.25, 500 at 1.30, 100 at 1.15, 1200 at 1.30.

Amulet—2000 at 1.75.

Siscoe—1300 at 65, 200 at 64, 500 at 62½, 50 at 61½, 1200 at 60, 500 at 55, 10,000 at 58, 1000 at 65.

Teck Hughes—500 at 5.10.

UNLISTED

Canadian Celanese Pfd.—75 at 42, 50 at 40.

Canada Malt—15 at 15, 50 at 16, 85 at 15, 10 at 14, 25 at 15.

Carlings—15 at 5¼, 100 at 3, 20 at 5.

Lake Superior—50 at 12, 75 at 11¼.

Perfection Glass—350 at 2.

UNLISTED OILS

Dalhousie Oil—30 at 1.75, 200 at 1.50.

Afternoon Transactions

Associated Breweries—85 at 21½, 295 at 21, 25 at 20½, 50 at 20¼, 50 at 20.

Associated Oil—290 at 1.20, 50 at 1.10, 3.50 at 1.00, 100 at .99, 325 at .95, 175 at 1.00, 170 at 1.10, 710 at 1.00, 80 at 1.25, 225 at 1.00, 115 at 1.10*, 200 at 1.25.

British American Oil—25 at 41, 20 at 40½, 150 at 40, 20 at 40¾, 360 at 41, 265 at 42, 25 at 41¾, 20 at 41½, 815 at 41, 115 at 40½, 595 at 40, 25 at 40⅞, 250 at 41, 125 at 41½, 90 at 42, 20 at 42½, 50 at 43, 105 at 41½, 45 at 41, 110 at 40½, 5 at 40¼, 90 at 40⅛, 130 at 40, 75 at 39, 110 at 40.

Commonwealth Pet.—1200 at 70, 100 at 75, 1000 at 65, 1200 at 70, 50 at 75.

Distillers-Seagrams—55 at 10¼, 50 at 10, 75 at 10½, 5 at 10¾, 75 at 10½, 125 at 10, 175 at 10½, 775 at 10, 25 at 10¼, 245 at 10, 70 at 10½, 10 at 10.

Dom. Eng. Works—125 at 65, 20 at 60.

Dryden Paper—25 at 17, 25 at 16½, 130 at 16, 20 at 16½, 15 at 17, 520 at 16½, 230 at 16.

Eastern Dairies—15 at 25, 50 at 20, 240 at 18, 25 at 17.

Foreign Securities—125 at 32, 50 at 31, 50 at 30.

Home Oil—20 at 11.50, 50 at 11.25, 75 at 10.00, 105 at 10.00, 35 at 10.50, 2170 at 10.00, 675 at 10.25.

Hydro Electric—100 at 38, 5 at 40, 25 at 35.

Imperial Tobacco—105 at 10, 600 at 9¾, 615 at 9½, 25 at 9¾, 130 at 9¼, 280 at 9, 120 at 9½, 20 at 10, 300 at 9¾.

Imperial Oil—18 at 29, 5 at 28¾, 70 at 28½, 100 at 28⅝, 550 at 28¼, 615 at 28, 5 at 26, 7 at 30, 244 at 29, 175 at 28½, 200 at 28¼, 300 at 28, 350 at 27¼, 555 at 27½, 5 at 27⅜, 390 at 27¼, 440 at 27, 75 at 26⅛, 325 at 26¾, 815 at 26½, 25 at 26⅜, 350 at 26¼, 485 at 26, 50 at 26¼, 420 at 26½, 175 at 26¾, 817 at 27, 25 at 26¼, 350 at 26¼, 605 at 26½, 575 at 26¼, 25 at 26½, 830 at 26, 5 at 25¾, 505 at 25, 200 at 25¼, 125 at 25½, 385 at 26, 320 at 34¼, 175 at 26½, 35 at 26¾, 35 at 26½, 200 at 26¼, 25 at 25⅜, 700 at 25, 10 at 25½, 125 at 25½, 230 at 25¾, 335 at 26, 10 at 26¼, 350 at 26½, 60 at 26¾, 335 at 28, 510 at 28¼, 150 at 28½, 240 at 28⅜, 300 at 28⅞, 1681 at 29, 260 at 29¼,

155 at 29½, 37 at 29*, 100 at 28¼, 500 at 28¾, 110 at 28⅝, 283 at 28½, 50 at 28¾, 220 at 28½, 601 at 28, 25 at 27¾, 100 at 27, 5 at 27½, 475 at 27¼.

Int. Petroleum—170 at 21, 50 at 20¼, 230 at 20½, 10 at 20¼, 795 at 20, 25 at 19¼, 25 at 19¾, 240 at 19½, 275 at 19, 15 at 18⅞, 100 at 19⅝, 280 at 19½, 110 at 19¾, 540 at 20, 110 at 20½, 630 at 21, 10 at 21¼, 160 at 21½, 295 at 20, 50 at 19¼, 50 at 19½, 410 at 19, 50 at 18½, 75 at 18¾, 800 at 18½, 200 at 18¾, 25 at 18⅞, 325 at 19, 225 at 19½, 415 at 19⅜, 25 at 19½, 260 at 20, 310 at 19¾, 200 at 19½, 1035 at 20, 25 at 20½, 20 at 19¾, 20 at 19½, 475 at 19, 100 at 19¾, 165 at 20.

Int. Petroleum—Continued—25 at 20¼, 275 at 20¾, 135 at 20½, 160 at 20¼, 25 at 20¼, 520 at 20, 115 at 19, 100 at 19⅛, 50 at 19¼, 45 at 19½, 75 at 19¾, 205 at 20.

International Paints—45 at 17.

Int. Utl. Class A—10 at 33, 50 at 33, 30 at 32, 35 at 32½, 35 at 31, 23 at 30, 55 at 31, 25 at 32, 25 at 31, 25 at 32, 10 at 31, 25 at 30, 25 at 29.

Int. Utl. class B—75 at 7, 5 at 8.

Manitoba Power—65 at 40, 5 at 39, 50 at 45.

Mitchell Robert—5 at 30.

Page-Hersey—25 at 90, 210 at 85, 5 at 84, 100 at 82, 130 at 80, 50 at 83, 10 at 84, 100 at 82.

Sarnia Bridge—Class B—50 at 12.

Walker—125 at 9, 175 at 9¼, 25 at 9½, 130 at 9, 100 at 9¼, 60 at 9, 145 at 8½, 60 at 9, 10 at 10, 280 at 9, 25 at 9¼, 80 at 9½, 325 at 10, 15 at 9¾, 150 at 9, 35 at 8½.

United Sec.—10 at 45.

Western Steel Products—55 at 35, 4 at 34, 25 at 33.

PREFERRED

Power Corp.—67 at 96, 40 at 95, 25 at 94.

S. Can. Power—50 at 105½.

United Sec.—16 at 103.

UNLISTED OILS

Dalhousie Oil—50 at 1.40, 450 at 1.50, 60 at 1.30, 150 at 1.20, 100 at 1.25, 235 at 1.10, 450 at 1.15.

Wainwell Oil—1,000 at 13, 7,000 at 11, 300 at 12½, 400 at 11, 500 at 14.

MINES

Abana—200 at 1.20, 300 at 1.18, 550 at 1.25, 400 at 1.20, 200 at 1.17, 100 at 1.15, 100 at 1.21, 5 at 1.40, 100 at 1.25, 550 at 1.20, 200 at 1.25.

Amulet—250 at 1.85.

Mining Corp.—200 at 2.80.

Noranda—210 at 25.50, 150 at 29.25, 25 at 28.75, 410 at 29.00, 25 at 29.25, 2 at 30.00, 190 at 29.00, 60 at 28.75, 660 at 28.50, 910 at 28.00, 300 at 27.75, 110 at 27.00, 615 at 27.50, 50 at 28.50, 630 at 28.00, 1,965 at 27.00, 100 at 26.50, 100 at 27.40, 1,505 at 27.50, 350 at 28.50, 200 at 30.00, 155 at 29.00, 392 at 30.00, 845 at 29.50, 515 at 29.25, 25 at 29.75, 2,175 at 29.00, 1,105 at 28.50, 35 at 28.00, 125 at 28.75, 210 at 28.90, 326 at 28.50, 185 at 29.00, 25 at 28.75, 230 at 28.00, 148 at 27.00, 125 at 26.75, 290 at 27.50.

Siscoe—500 at .58, 200 at .53, 300 at .60, 1,800 at 55, 100 at .50, 50 at .58, 1,250 at .55, 7,700 at .51, 1,900 at .50, 1,500 at .55.

Teck Hughes—600 at 5.00, 450 at 4.75.

UNLISTED

Canadian Celanese pfd.—10 at 41, 25 at 40.

Canada Malt—10 at 14, 5 at 12, 10 at 13, 135 at 12, 120 at 13, 90 at 12, 50 at 11½, 40 at 15, 25 at 15½, 260 at 16, 100 at 17¼, 100 at 17½, 10 at 15.

Carlings—100 at 2, 10 at 3½, 65 at 4, 50 at 4.

Lake Superior—25 at 11¼, 110 at 7, 100 at 10, 25 at 8½, 100 at 8, 65 at 7, 70 at 8½, 570 at 10.

Perfection Glass—340 at 2.

(From the *Gazette*, October 30, 1929.)

Index

Gold Diggers of 1929

General Electric, 45

General Motors, 70, 71

Germany, 2, 61

Goforth, William W., 96

gold. See mining and mining speculation

Gooderham, George, 42

Goodyear Tire and Rubber, 113

Gordon, Sir Charles, 42

grain and grain speculation, 51–63, 68–9, 78, 114; effect of Crash on, 61–3, 74, 97, 102, 114

grain exchanges, 56–9. See also under individual cities

Gray, James H., 35, 57, 60

Great Depression. See Depression

Greenshields, 23

Guaranty Trust, 99

Guelph Daily Mercury, 74

Guelph, Ontario, 66, 71–3

Hammell, Jack, 27

Harper's, 140

Harvard Economic Society, 38

Hatch, H. C., 83

Hatry, Clarence, 95

Heppleston, James, 33

Hershey Chocolate, 116

Hill, James J., 66

Hiram Walker-Gooderham and Worts, 83, 96

Hollinger Mines, 35

Holt, Sir Herbert, 6, 66, 88, 90, 113

Home Bank of Canada, 9, 88

Homer L. Gibson and Company, 33

Hoover, Herbert, 103

Horn, Michiel, 128–9

Horne, Edmund, 24

Houde, Camillien, 22

House of Morgan. See J. P. Morgan and Company

Howard Smith Paper, 89

Hudson Bay Mining and Smelting, 35

Hunnings, H. E., 30

Hush, 91

Imperial Bank, 115

Imperial Oil, 45

India, 62

International Harvester, 38

International Nickel, 45, 84, 96, 101, 106, 107, 111, 117

investment trusts, 18–20, 38, 99

Italy, 61

J. P. Morgan and Company, 99, 100, 105, 106

Jolliffe, Col. W. H., 94

Kennedy, Joseph, 41, 116

Keynes, John Maynard, 3, 136–7

Killam, Izaak Walton, 88

King, W. L. Mackenzie, 7, 14–5, 16, 51, 83, 132

Kingston, Ontario, 16, 33

Kirkland Lake, Ontario, 24

Kitchener, Ontario, 128

Knowles, R. E., 77, 120, 121

Kraft Cheese, 166

Kreuger, Ivar, 5

Lamont, Thomas W., 99

Larkin, P. C., 14, 83

Leacock, Stephen, 22

Lennox, E. J., 89

Liberal Party, 7, 132

Lingle, Jake, 68

Livermore, Jesse L., 74, 104

Loblaws, 98, 116

Logan, S. H., 115

Longbottom, Ralph, 108

Lougheed, Sir James, 15, 52

Macdonald, Ross, 127

Mackenzie, A. B., 103

Maclean, Col. John B., 15

Malone, Richard S., 62–3

Manitoba, 32, 35, 53, 59

Manitoba Pool Elevators, 54

Marshall, Benjamin, 72

Martin, Médéric, 113

Massey-Harris, 40, 98

Mauff, John R., 78

Meggeson, Jack, 105

Mellon, Andrew, 37

Michaelovich, Grand Duke Alexandr, 93

Miller, S. W., 85, 86

Mills, Harvey, 31, 33

mining and mining speculation, 24–6, 29; copper (Noranda), 20, 45, 96, 118, 133; fraud in, 20, 21–2, 24–5, 26–8, 30–5, 133–4; gold, 34, 35, 41; Manitoba, 35; Montreal and Quebec, 22, 35, 91, 133, 134; nickel (International Nickel), 84, 96, 101, 106, 107, 111, 117; silver, 24, 91; Toronto and Ontario, 24, 35, 91–2, 131, 132, 133. See also Standard Stock and Mining Exchange

Mitchell, Charles E., 99, 105

Monetary Times, 29

Montgomery Ward, 16, 38, 70, 76

Montreal, 22–4, 45, 48, 84, 86, 88, 91, 93, 124, 131, 132, 133

Montreal Curb Exchange, 21, 98

Montreal Gazette, 17, 45–6, 47, 48, 91, 92, 102, 113

Montreal Light, Heat and Power, 88, 101

Montreal Star, 91, 122